The Apple Vinegar Complete Guide & recipes for Numerous Health Conditions, using ACV Miracle Health System

Regina Williams

Copyright © 2020 Regina Williams

All rights reserved. No part of this publication may be reproduced, distributed, or transmitted in any form or by any means, including photocopying, recording, or other electronic or mechanical methods, without the prior written permission of the publisher, except in the case of brief quotations embodied in critical reviews and specific other non-commercial uses permitted by copyright law.

ISBN: 978-1-63750-179-5

Table of Contents

THE APPLE CIDER VINEGAR COMPLETE GUIDE & RECIPES FOR NUMEROUS HEALTH CONDITIONS, USING ACV MIRACLE HEALTH SYSTEM I

INTRODUCTION 8

CHAPTER 1 11

WHAT IS APPLE CIDER VINEGAR? 11
WHAT IS "THE MOTHER" IN APPLE CIDER VINEGAR? 18
THE ORIGIN OF APPLE CIDER VINEGAR? 19
THE TAKEAWAY 25
DOES APPLE CIDER VINEGAR CAUSE DIARRHEA? 27
APPLE CIDER VINEGAR FOR WARTS 27
    Effectiveness of ACV to Wart 28
    ACV Step-by-Step Guide for Wart 29
    ACV Step-by-Step Guide for Weightloss 30
    Bottom line 32
APPLE CIDER VINEGAR CLEANSING 33
    Fast Facts about the ACV Detox 34
    Great Things about an ACV Detox 34
APPLE CIDER VINEGAR FOR PSORIASIS 35
HOW TO TAKE APPLE CIDER VINEGAR 37

CHAPTER 2 42

CONSTITUENTS OF ACV 42
TYPES OF APPLE CIDER VINEGAR 43
    Raw Apple Cider Vinegar 43
    Pasteurized Apple Cider Vinegar 44
APPLE CIDER VINEGAR AND ACID REFLUX DISORDER 46
APPLE CIDER VINEGAR AND WEIGHTLOSS 50
APPLE CIDER VINEGAR FOR THE HAIR 53
APPLE CIDER VINEGAR FOR SKIN 60
HEALTH BENEFITS OF ORGANIC ACV 66
    Blood Sugar 66
    Weight Loss 67
HOW TO USE APPLE CIDER VINEGAR IN YOUR DAILY DIET 68

Salad Dressing... 68
Probiotic Tonic 68
Marinade 69
Cocktails or drinks 69
OTHER USES OF ACV 69
Dandruff.. 70
Dry Scalp Sunburn along with other Skin Injuries 70
Acne and other Chronic Skin Disorders 71
Sore Throat 72
Deodorant for Smelly Feet 73
IS APPLE CIDER VINEGAR SAFE?... 74
SIDE EFFECTS OF ACV... 75
DOSAGE AND PREPARATION.. 77
METHODS FOR SAFE USE OF ACV 80

CHAPTER 3 83

HOUSEHOLD BENEFITS OF APPLE CIDER VINEGAR.. 83
Being a cleansing agent... 83
Remove oil from pots and pans 84
Cleaning Windows 84
Removing stains from your carpet.. 85
Removing lime build-up 85
Deodorizing your house 86
Keeping ants away... 86
Prevent fading of clothes 87
Prevent the formation of ice in your windshield 87
Removing Wall Paper 88
Flowers and Grass.. 88

CHAPTER 4 89

APPLE CIDER VINEGAR FOR HEALING NUMEROUS HEALTH CONDITIONS 89
Problems with Potassium Deficiency 90
APPLE CIDER VINEGAR FOR BODY CLEANSING.. 92
APPLE CIDER VINEGAR RELIEVES HEADACHES 93

iv

- ACV Improves Weight Loss Greatly 96
- Fast Body Metabolism 97
- Suppress Your Appetite 98
- Help Intermittent Fasting 100
- Detoxify Your Liver 102
- Gallbladder Cleansing 104
- Calm Heartburn 105
- Reduce Flatulence 107
- Soothe stomachaches 109
- Alleviate pregnancy morning sickness 110
- Relieve bouts of constipation 112
- Overcome Diarrhea 114
- Avoid Bacterial Cystitis (UTI) 116
- Limit Interstitial Cystitis 118
- Minimize Iron Insufficiency 119
- Increase Calcium Absorption 121
- Avoid Vitamin C Deficiencies 123
- Avoid Vitamin-B Deficiencies 125
- Irritable Bowel Syndrome (IBS) 129
- Enhance a Vegetarian Diet Plan 131

CHAPTER 5 133

- ACV For Complete Wellness 133
  - *Detoxify The Natural Way* 135
  - *Improve A Diabetic Lifestyle* 137
  - *Help Safeguard against Cancer* 139
  - *End The Hiccups* 141
  - *Relieve Muscle Stiffness* 143
  - *Get Rid of a Stuffy Nose* 144
  - *Ease a Sore Throat* 146
  - *Soothe Sinusitis* 147
  - *Combat High Cholesterol* 149
  - *Reduce Bad Breath* 151
  - *Fight Exhaustion* 153
  - *Overcome Laryngitis* 155

Relieve Leg Pain 157
Reduces the Chance of Cataracts 159
Alleviate Foot Fungus 161
Reduce Asthma Symptoms 162
Reduce Swelling 164
Whitening of Teeth 166
Resolves renal issues 167
Exercise Daily 169

CHAPTER 6 171
HONEY & APPLE CIDER VINEGAR 171
POTENTIAL BENEFITS OF ACV & HONEY 172
Acetic acid promote weight-loss 172
Help alleviate seasonal allergies and cold symptoms 173
Improves heart health 174
Potential downside 175
Possible effects on blood sugar levels and cholesterol 175
Could be harsh on your stomach and teeth 176
Can be saturated in sugar 176
Purported effects on body alkalinity 177
BEST USES OF ACV 178

CHAPTER 7 181
APPLE CIDER VINEGAR FOR HAIR CARE 181
Help Hair Thinning 183
Make Your Hair Rinse 185
Produce Your Shampoo 186
Produce Your Conditioner 188
Combat Baldness 189
Detangle Hair 191
Reduce Frizz 192
Prevent Split Ends 194
Kill and Stop Headlice 196
Promote Hair Regrowth 197

Remove Hard Water Residue *199*

Add Shine *200*

Highlight Hair *202*

Drive Back Chlorine Damage *203*

Promote Scalp Health *205*

Remove Product Residue *206*

CHAPTER 8 .... **209**

APPLE CIDER VINEGAR FOR SKIN CARE 209

Cleanse Your Pores *211*

Tone Your Skin Layer *212*

Minimize Psoriasis *214*

Ease Sunburn *216*

Remove Acne *218*

Diminish Eczema *220*

Soothe Diaper Rash *222*

Relieve Hemorrhoids *223*

Relieve Insect Bites *225*

Mitigate Jellyfish Stings *227*

Decrease the Exposure to Facial "Masks" *228*

Lessen Age Spots *230*

Counteract Varicose Veins *232*

Manage Nail Fungus *234*

Cleanse and Push away Infection from Cuts *235*

Produce Your Own Deodorant *237*

CHAPTER 9 .... **240**

SIDE EFFECTS OF APPLE CIDER VINEGAR 240

Reduced potassium levels *240*

Digestive issues *240*

Interactions with other medication *241*

Damaged tooth enamel *241*

CHAPTER 10 .... **242**

HOW TO MAKE ACV FROM HOME 242

PRECAUTIONS 244

Introduction

Do you want to learn the recipes and step-by-step guide for healing numerous health conditions, using ACV Miracle Health System?

The use of Organic Apple Cider Vinegar is a wonderful health aid, and the *#1* food and home essential I recommend in helping to maintain the body's vital acid-alkaline balance.

The natural, undistilled Apple Cider Vinegar (ACV) is a powerful cleansing and healing elixir, *"a naturally occurring antibiotic and antiseptic that fights germs and bacteria"* for a healthier, stronger, and longer life!

The book is your ultimate guide to using apple cider vinegar for healing various health conditions. You'll discover recipes for treating many health conditions, from trivial cases to some severe diseases such as diabetes, blood sugar level control, weight loss, heart health, liver cleansing, and many more.

In this book, you will learn all of the science-backed, information about raw organic, unfiltered, and unpasteurized apple cider vinegar for various use which includes;

- Detoxifying the liver, kidney, and lungs,
- How to use Apple Cider Vinegar for removing *wart*, losing weight, and reduce blood sugar level with step-by-step instructions,
- The usefulness of ACV and Honey for various purposes,
- How to use Apple Cider Vinegar for healing several health conditions such as; headaches, weight-loss, fast metabolism, gall bladder cleansing, heartburn, stomachaches, diarrhea, bacterial cystitis (UTI), detoxifying liver, pregnancy morning sickness, irritable bowel syndrome (IBS),
- How to use Apple Cider Vinegar for enhancing a vegetarian diet plan,
- How to improve bad breath, relieve asthma symptoms and improve diabetic lifestyle,
- How to make Apple cider vinegar from home,
- For easing sunburn, toning skin, soothe diaper rash, relieve insect bites, lesson age spots, remove acne, cleanse pores, diminish eczema,
- How to make Mother Nature's All-in-one, All-Natural, Cure-all, and Multi-purpose Miracle Health System - Apple Cider Vinegar from home

with step-by-step instruction.

…and lot more.

Apple cider vinegar is a naturally occurring antibiotic and antiseptic that fights germs and bacteria for a healthier, stronger, and longer life!

Chapter 1
What is Apple Cider Vinegar?

People have used apple cider vinegar medicinally and therapeutically for several years, and currently, it's prevalent. Beware of the hype, not every claim concerning this product holds. In this book, you will learn all of the science-backed, vetted great things about raw, organic, unfiltered, and unpasteurized apple cider vinegar.

ACV is "a naturally occurring antibiotic and antiseptic that fights germs and bacteria" for a healthier, stronger, longer life!

The versatility of ACV as a powerful body cleansing agent is legendary.

It's best for your gut

The fermentation process that yields apple cider vinegar encourages the growth and proliferation of good-for-your-gut microbes. Consuming probiotic-rich fermented foods offers is shown to *boost digestion, raise the immune system, as well as positively affect mental health*. A lot of the probiotics in apple cider vinegar are within the cloudy **"mother"** strands you will discover floating in it, so make sure to buy apple cider vinegar that still has the *mother* intact.

Beyond being filled with probiotics, *apple cider vinegar are advantageous for gut health.* As functional medicine practitioner Will Cole, D.C., IFMCP, explains, *"apple cider vinegar, also, has been shown to have antiviral and anti-yeast and antifungal benefits, all helpful in supporting microbiome and overall immune balance."*

It controls blood sugar levels

Apple cider vinegar can help combat that spike-then-crash blood glucose roller coaster you can feel following a carb-heavy meal. In a single small study, supplementing a higher glycemic meal (think a bagel and juice) with apple cider vinegar reduced post-meal blood sugar by about 50% in healthy patients. In a twin study from the same authors, participants with diabetes or insulin resistance saw blood-sugar-balancing advantages from ACV as well.

So before digging into the starchy faves like pasta, potatoes, and pretzels, try sipping on just a little apple cider vinegar.

It can assist in weight loss

Among apple cider vinegar's best-known benefits is its role in weight loss. While there have never been many reports on ACV and weight maintenance, there were studies on its components, like acetic acid. In a report of obese Japanese adults, it had been discovered that subjects who consumed acetic acid for 12 weeks experienced significant weight reduction and declines in belly fat, waist circumference, and triglycerides in comparison to those that consumed a placebo.

Researchers believe it functions by suppressing appetite. Acetic acid has been proven to delay gastric emptying, meaning you are feeling fuller for longer. That is likely why apple cider vinegar consumption, also, has been weakly connected with the lower total energy consumption during the day.

While further research is necessary, you may safely include ACV within a healthy weight reduction routine. Make an effort adding 2 teaspoons of apple cider vinegar to 16 ounces of water and sipping this concoction each day.

Apple cider vinegar has antibacterial, antifungal, and antiviral properties, and that means you may use it to completely clean from your kitchen floor, bathroom, and many more.

Just mix half a cup of apple cider vinegar with a cup of water, and get cleaning. Utilize this solution to completely clean microwaves, kitchen surfaces, windows, glasses, and mirrors. *It is also found in dishwashers as an alternative for dish detergent.*

Apple cider vinegar will clean your toilets and leave your bathrooms smelling like apples.

Through the use of apple cider vinegar instead of additional products, you could decrease the usage of severe chemicals in your house and lifestyle.

You can use it to clean products.

Even though your produce is organic, there can be pesticides. Apple cider vinegar is a superb way to clean those off and eradicate any germs from your fruits and veggies. *Research shows that ACV reduces the amount of Salmonella bacteria on fresh salad vegetables*. To improve the bacteria-fighting powers, mix in lemon juice, as this combination was found to become exceptionally effective.

It can produce your hair shine

Your scalp and hair's natural pH is just about 5.5, rendering it acidic. The regular shampoo is alkaline, that may toss off your hair's pH, causing brittle, dry strands. Water, too, can transform the hair's pH, since water's pH is usually neutral. Apple cider vinegar's acidity helps it be an ideal post-shampoo rinse to help significantly restore pH balance, boosting hair's shine and health.

Try recycling a vintage shampoo bottle, then filling it with ½ tablespoon of apple cider vinegar and 1 cup of lukewarm water. Pour the perfect solution through your hair after shampooing.

Bonus: ACV can help remove flaky dandruff. As a result of its antifungal houses, it could work against a number of the common factors behind dandruff, just like a build-up of oil or perhaps a yeast-like fungus called *Malassezia*.

It can be a skin toner

The acidity and anti-inflammatory nature of ACV make it an excellent addition to your skin layer care routine. Dilute it with two parts water, and spread the concoction over that person having a cotton ball to displace your present toner. You can do this during the night after washing and each day before you apply your moisturizer. The acidity helps slough away dead skin cells while soothing irritation.

It's essential to notice that because of its acidic nature, apple cider vinegar alone could cause skin irritation. Always dilute apple cider vinegar before using topically.

It could remove stains from teeth

Make an effort mixing two parts apple cider vinegar and one part baking soda for an all-natural tooth-whitening paste. Rub teeth directly using the apple cider vinegar paste and rinse with water. The results will not be immediate but done several times a week; this will help remove stains and whiten teeth. You can even gargle with ACV for an identical effect.

Bonus: Gargling apple cider vinegar will relieve bad breath. Its antibacterial properties can kill stinky breath bacteria. It's worth noting that, because of its acidity, there is certainly some concern that consuming ACV can contribute to tooth enamel decay, just like soda and fruit drinks do. So we advise caution with this technique and do not recommend carrying it out long term.

It could repel fleas from your pets

While apple cider vinegar won't necessarily rid your dog of the flea problem, it can prevent one. Fleas don't like the smell or taste of Vinegar so that ACV could be a sound natural repellent.

Make an effort spraying one part vinegar and one part water on your own pet's fur and rubbing it in generously.

Saturate the complete coat, and continue each day for a couple of days to weekly.

What is "the Mother" in Apple Cider Vinegar?

Apple cider vinegar is manufactured out of apple juice, and it is fermented to hard apple cider. It's then fermented another time to be *apple cider vinegar*. In large volumes, it is recognized to contain *vitamins, minerals, proteins, organic acids (acetic acid and citric acid), and polyphenolic compounds (micronutrients are known to function in the prevention of disease).*

When apple cider vinegar is manufactured utilizing a slow fermentation process, there's a build-up of yeast and bacteria. This build-up, called ***the mother***, is often considered to contain a lot of essential ingredients *(enzymes and proteins)*. The mother helps it appear slightly cloudy and could even arrive in strands or sediment inside the finished product. When buying, you always want to get one using the mother still intact, as this is the area of the Vinegar that retains lots of the beneficial ingredients. Be sure you shake it well to disperse the mother before you utilize it.

The Origin of Apple Cider Vinegar?

Vinegar originates from the French phrase *vin aigre*, meaning sour wine. The sourness originates from the acetic acid. Making apple cider vinegar entails benefiting from controlled-spoilage.

Yeast digests the sugars in apples and converts them into alcohol. A bacteria, *acetobacter*, then turns the alcohol into acetic acid. I don't need to get too technical; nevertheless, you can call this technique fermentation. The ***"mother"*** identifies the mix of yeast and bacteria formed during fermentation. If you take a look at an apple cider vinegar bottle, you can view strands of the *"mother"* going swimming.

Many people attribute apple cider vinegar's effects on the *"mother."* There's some truth to this because the mother counts like a probiotic. But, the need for the mother is not established with research. Apart from probiotics, ACV includes a vitamin profile similar to apple juice. Hence, the sour drink is ripe with B-vitamins and polyphenols (plant-based antioxidants).

Overall, the probiotics, acetic acid, as well as the nutrients in ACV are in charge of its health advantages. ACV may have a modest influence on weight loss, but don't remove your gym membership.

Apple cider vinegar helps with blood sugar control.
It's no secret that diabetes is common in America. Is ACV an acceptable weapon to fight diabetes?

It is, according to some studies. One of these is a little study published Journal with the American Association of Diabetes in 2004. The analysis entailed giving participants meals made up of a bagel, OJ, and butter. Following the meal, the participants received 20 grams of apple cider vinegar or even a placebo. The researchers checked blood sugar amounts 30 and 60 minutes following the meal.

They discovered that ACV significantly lowered post-meal blood sugar levels. Other studies report similar findings.

Important Note: ACV won't cure diabetes; however, it may moderately lower blood sugar levels. It won't consider the area of any medications for diabetes; however, it's a safe addition to a diabetes treatment solution (so long as you don't have kidney disease).

Apple cider vinegar may keep the bacteria carefully on your salad from getting out from control.

In 2005, a report assessed Vinegar's anti-microbial properties by inoculating arugula with *Salmonella*. The researchers treated the tainted arugula with either Vinegar, lemon juice, or a combined mix of them both. The researchers sought to see if these interventions could reduce bacterial growth. They discovered that both lemon juice and Vinegar decreased the growth of *Salmonella*. The ACV/lemon juice mixture decreased *Salmonella* to undetectable levels (I wouldn't bank on this in the home, though).

Important Note: *Nowadays, it looks like there's a recall for lettuces at least one time each week. Throwing some ACV on the salad may serve a purpose beyond adding flavor. Even though you use ACV, you've still got to use good sense. In case you dip raw chicken within your spinach, the Vinegar won't stop the bout of diarrhea that's coming.*

Apple cider vinegar can help boost weight-loss.

Everyone wants to slim down. Supplements that facilitate weight loss are popular. And since it works out, a randomized, clinical trial recently published in the Journal of Functional Food showed that ACV would help with weight loss.

The participants drank 15ml of ACV with lunch and dinner (a complete of 2 tablespoons). In addition, they ate a diet that was 250 calories significantly less than their day-by-day approximated requirements. The researchers discovered that ACV considerably reduced weight. The people in the ACV group typically lost 8.8 lbs over 12 weeks. Alternatively, the participants who didn't receive

ACV just lost 5 pounds over the 12 week study period. The researchers also discovered that ACV reduced cholesterol levels.

Important Note: *ACV may have a modest influence on weight reduction, but don't remove your gym membership. Take into account that the people with this report were on the calorie-restricted diet plus they exercised. The researchers argued that ACV affects weight by lowering one's appetite.*

Apple cider vinegar won't control your high blood pressure.

One popular myth is the fact that ACV could be utilized for controlling blood pressure. In my research, I came across one small study in rats that showed a reduction in systolic blood pressure when fed with a diet plan containing acetic acid in comparison to those without it. There weren't any studies using ACV for high blood pressure in people.

Important Note: *High blood pressure is usually nothing to play with. I've seen people who have strokes in real-*

time from high blood pressure. When you have high blood pressure, there's not enough data to aid using ACV like a blood pressure medication. Eat a nutritious diet, exercise, and take your meds if you have them.

Apple cider vinegar will not cure cancer.

A few studies also show that Vinegar may have anti-cancer properties. Many of these studies involved culturing cancer cells and exposing these to Vinegar or acetic acid. The restriction of the studies is apparent; we can't directly pour ACV on cancers within people. Further, you certainly can't give someone an ACV IV infusion without causing severe harm or death.

Yet, a significant population study from China found lower rates of esophageal cancer in individuals who frequently consumed Vinegar. It's worth noting that the people in the analysis were most likely consuming rice vinegar, not ACV.

Important Note: *ACV won't cure esophageal cancer, unfortunately. Like a GI doctor, I'm usually the first* *person to inform someone that he or she has got esophageal cancer. I possibly could tell people all they need to do is drink some vinegar. Sadly, things aren't that simple. If you're concerned about the chance of esophageal cancer, then don't smoke and don't drink a whole lot of alcohol. Speak to your doctor when you have chronic heartburn because you might need screening for Barrett's esophagus.*

The takeaway

Generally, ACV is safe. Everything includes a possible downside, even ACV. Before you begin guzzling apple cider vinegar, here are some negative possibilities. The acid in apple cider vinegar may erode your enamel; you might guzzle some normal water after drinking it. Anecdotally, acidic foods or liquids like Vinegar may exacerbate acid reflux disorder.

When you have chronic kidney disease, your kidneys may possibly not be able to operate the surplus acid that comes along with drinking apple cider vinegar.

Like any supplement, ACV won't replace a wholesome lifestyle. It could have some advantages to our anatomies.

However, overall, we need more studies to understand medical benefits and unwanted effects connected with ACV seriously. Apple cider vinegar is becoming popular as an all-natural remedy for several ailments.

Did it cause diarrhea, or might it be utilized to take care of it?

Apple cider vinegar could be found in cooking, taken as a pill, or coupled with water. Since it is quite acidic, it could cause stomach discomfort or digestive problems. However, that is unlikely to occur unless a person drinks a substantial amount on the undiluted Vinegar.

Research into apple cider vinegar is bound; however, many people do experience unwanted adverse effects. Furthermore, to diarrhea, these effects include harm to tooth enamel and stomach problems in people who have diabetes.

Does Apple Cider Vinegar cause Diarrhea?

Acidic foods could cause an upset stomach or diarrhea.

Apple cider vinegar is manufactured by fermenting the sugar in apples. The fermentation process creates acetic acid, the main elemental part of Vinegar that means it is acidic. Some individuals could find that acidic or spicy foods could cause an upset stomach, heartburn, or diarrhea.

Infections such as food poisoning are typical factors behind diarrhea. Food allergies or certain medical conditions, such as celiac disease or irritable bowel syndrome, may also cause diarrhea.

Apple Cider Vinegar for Warts

Many treatments are available to warts, including removal by a health care provider, over-the-counter medication, and home cures, such as apple cider vinegar. Warts are rough bumps of the skin due to the *human papillomavirus (HPV)*. Apple cider vinegar's effectiveness for treating warts isn't known, and there are reports of risks and complications with this *do-it-yourself* solution.

We shall take a close look at what sort of person might use apple cider vinegar on warts, its effectiveness, and unwanted effects. We would also talk about different ways to take care of warts.

Effectiveness of ACV to Wart

Apple cider vinegar on the table could be useful for warts
Vinegar enables you to kill some bacteria, but apple cider vinegar is not tested for this function.

There happens to be no scientific research to claim that apple cider vinegar is an efficient treatment for warts.

The theory behind this treatment would be that the acid should destroy the wart tissue, similar to what *salicylic acid does. At high concentrations, salicylic acid could be more effective when compared to a placebo for treating warts.*

Generally, Vinegar may be used to kill some types of bacteria. According to one study, Vinegar could be effective against common bacteria, including *Escherichia coli (E. Coli) and Salmonella*. However, scientists never have tested this theory with *apple cider vinegar*.

There can also be some unwanted effects of using acidic products on your skin, so a person considering this treatment should proceed with caution. Apple cider vinegar is available in many food markets and online.

ACV Step-by-Step Guide for Wart

When working with apple cider vinegar to take care of a wart, an individual can follow these steps:

- ✓ Gather a bottle of apple cider vinegar, cotton balls or cotton-tipped applicators, and a little bandage.
- ✓ Soak the cotton ball in apple cider vinegar and apply this to the region where in fact, the wart is.
- ✓ Place the bandage on the cotton ball and leave it set up overnight. Some individuals may leave it on for 24 hours.
- ✓ Replace the cotton ball with a brand new one dipped in apple cider vinegar every night.

The wart may swell or throb. Your skin in the wart risk is turning black within the first one to two days, which can signal that your skin cells inside the wart are dying.

The wart might fall off within 14 days. Continuing to utilize apple cider vinegar to get a few days following this may avoid the skin cells that caused the prior wart from shedding and growing elsewhere.

ACV Step-by-Step Guide for Weightloss

The internet wants to gush on using apple cider vinegar for weight loss. If weight reduction is an objective for you, ACV can impact both weight and surplus fat. Wanting to slim down is okay, but remember - you're an ideal ray of *#WokeUpLikeThis* awesomeness just when you are. Here's the DL:

A Japanese study from 2009 divided several adults with obesity into three groups.

For 12 weeks, one group took 1 tablespoon (15 milliliters) of ACV every day, the next group took 2 tablespoons (30 milliliters) of ACV, and the third group took a placebo.

The common benefits observed from the first group (who consumed 1 tablespoon of ACV each day) were:
- ✓ 2.6 pounds of weight lost
- ✓ 0.7% reduction in body fat
- ✓ 0.5-inch reduction in waist circumference
- ✓ 25% reduction in triglycerides.

The common benefits for the next group (who consumed 2 tablespoons of ACV each day) were:
- ✓ 3.7 pounds of weight lost
- ✓ 0.9% reduction in body fat
- ✓ 0.75-inch reduction in waist circumference
- ✓ 26% reduction in triglycerides

The placebo group gained typically 0.9 pounds, and their waist circumference increased slightly.

Just a few human studies have investigated ACV's relationship to weight reduction, so while this study is significant, we need even more research to feel good about it.

In another 2009 examination, mice were fed a higher fat, high-calorie diet for 6 weeks. Much like the human study, these were split into three groups: an organization that received a minimal dose of ACV. An organization received a higher dose of ACV and a control group.

By the end of 6 weeks, the group finding a high dose of ACV had gained 10% less fat compared to the control group. They'd also gained 2% less fat compared to the group that received a lesser dose of ACV. These details are pretty rad, but we'll need more conclusive info before breaking out the ticker tape.

Bottom line

Research shows that a regular dose of 1-2 tablespoons of apple cider vinegar could assist in weight loss and decrease the surplus fat percentage, stomach fat, and blood triglycerides. *Honey and Vinegar* have already been utilized for medicinal and culinary purposes for a large number of years, with people often combining both like a health tonic.

The mixture, which is usually diluted with water, is considered to provide a selection of health advantages, including weight loss and reduced blood sugar. For years, people have tried to look for the best methods to shed pounds and achieve a wholesome, fit, and trim appearance. You will find multiple reasons why weight reduction is really a recommended and healthy pursuit. Extra fat can contribute to a number of problems including oily skin and hair, unhealthy strain on the bones and joints, an elevated risk of cardiovascular disease and diabetes as well as premature death. The simple truth is, the overall state of American health has been around a perpetually declining trend for many years. Individuals who wish to discover a- *'without headaches'* way to lose excess weight will likely exist disappointed, as there is absolutely no magic bullet. People who are ready to work to lose weight but remain longing for an ally that will aid them in their weight reduction journey to create their efforts far better could find apple cider vinegar to become a perfect option.

Apple Cider Vinegar Cleansing

During the last couple of years, cleansing diets have already been growing steadily in popularity. One of these detox diets involves using apple cider vinegar - an amber-colored vinegar created from cider or apple must.

Testifiers to the *apple cider vinegar (ACV)* detox say it can help with fat loss, removal of toxins from your body, and blood glucose regulation. Despite many anecdotal success stories, little scientific evidence exists to aid these claims. Read on to find more about the ACV detox, including how exactly to follow the dietary plan plus the potential unwanted effects a person may experience.

Fast Facts about the ACV Detox

There isn't much research to claim that any kind of *"cleanse"* can detoxify your body completely.

A simple ACV detox involves consuming the Vinegar about three times a day. Trying an ACV cleansing over a short-term basis is probably safe for many people.

Great Things about an ACV Detox

Apple cider vinegar includes several purported benefits, including aiding weight-loss.

Proponents in the ACV diet say that consuming ACV, either daily or within an ardent ACV detox, brings the following benefits:

- *Helping with weight reduction*
- *Reducing appetite*
- *Balancing the body's pH*
- *Regulating blood sugar*
- *Lowering raised cholesterol*
- *Improving digestion*
- *Boosting the disease fighting capability*
- *Providing probiotics (high bacteria) for the gut*
- *Aiding in removing toxins*
- *Healing skin conditions*
- *Providing enzymes to your body.*

Some individuals may undertake an ACV detox to kick-start a wholesome lifestyle, filled with a far more balanced diet and regular physical exercise.

Apple Cider Vinegar for Psoriasis

Psoriasis can be a condition that triggers thick, scaly, and reddened patches to seem on your skin. Some people think that apple cider vinegar might help alleviate the itching and irritation that psoriasis often causes.

Psoriasis will not yet have a remedy, but there are numerous treatments and medications available that will help people manage their symptoms. While conventional medications, such as steroid creams, might help ease the symptoms, many people choose to use home cures, such as apple cider vinegar.

The above information examines apple cider vinegar being a psoriasis treatment, including its benefits and risks. We also check out different natural choices to take care of psoriasis. Apple cider vinegar will help soothe some symptoms of psoriasis.

Due to its antiseptic properties, apple cider vinegar can help soothe the itching or irritation from psoriasis, especially for the scalp, based on the National Psoriasis Foundation.

Those who sustain its use suggest applying the vinegar right to the scalp many times a week. Some individuals report seeing a noticeable difference within their condition within a couple of weeks. However, when the scalp can be cracked, bleeding, or if you find open wounds, apple cider vinegar will probably cause further irritation and pain.

Vinegar could cause a burning sensation, so moderating the dose would be ideal for avoiding further irritation.

Diluting the Vinegar with equal levels of water before putting it on can also decrease the sensation of burning and irritation. Rinsing the scalp after the solution has dried could also alleviate these effects. Although there look like no risks when working with apple cider vinegar for psoriasis, no direct research has determined its effects on the problem.

How to Take Apple Cider Vinegar.

Step 1

Find out about the nutrition info and chemical composition of apple cider vinegar to be able to determine how this supplement could work on healthy weight loss.

Apple cider vinegar can be an acidic liquid that's created from the fermentation of whole apples. The science behind apple cider vinegar as a highly effective weight loss supplement is questioned in lots of academic circles. You can find, however, the same number of nutritionists and dietitians who think that apple cider vinegar can curb appetite and promote gradual fat burning.

Step 2

Understand what to consider when purchasing apple cider vinegar. Many apple cider vinegar products are distilled way too many times. Each distillation or filtration process strips the apple cider vinegar of essential nutrients and vitamins.

Purchase apple cider vinegar or apple cider vinegar supplements that are produced from whole apples that avoid Vinegar that is distilled or filtered.

Step 3

Purchase apple cider vinegar from a health grocery instead of from a supermarket. This will make sure that the Vinegar you are purchasing still includes all the positive characteristics of the weight loss supplement instead of apple cider vinegar that's designed simply for cooking.

Step 4

Consume one to two teaspoons of apple cider vinegar before every single meal. Some consumers choose to dilute the apple cider vinegar within an 8-ounce glass of water or iced tea.

When the flavor of apple cider vinegar is too strong for you to consume frequently comfortably, you might choose to include one to two teaspoons of raw honey to some dose of apple cider vinegar.

Step 5

Use a journal that catalogs your usage of apple cider vinegar as well as your levels of energy, food cravings, appetite spikes, sleeping habits, and fat loss. Within your journal, list the quantity of apple cider vinegar you used before meals, the method where you consumed the apple cider vinegar, as well as the meal which you followed your dose with.

Compare these facts with your leads to determine which kind of apple cider vinegar does is most reliable for the body.

Step 6

Understand that effective fat loss is virtually impossible if the number of calories you are burning every day will not exceed the number of calories that you will be consuming every day. While apple cider vinegar can help limit your appetite and increase your metabolism, you won't replace the necessity for a fitness regimen and a healthy diet plan. Just by pairing healthy eating with regular aerobic exercise, you will be able to slim down over time.

Step 7

Be patient in regards to the weight-loss effects of apple cider vinegar. Apple cider vinegar isn't a miracle drug; actually, no such miracle drug exists. The only path to lose excess weight within an effective and healthy way is usually to take action gradually, giving your fat cells period to regulate and adjust to their new size.

Apple cider vinegar is considered to increase weight reduction by about fifteen pounds every year. An additional fifteen pounds of fat loss each year could make an enormous difference in one's appearance and general health.

Step 8

Calculate the body mass index and regulate how much weight you will need to reduce to accomplish your ideal weight. Set specific weight loss goals on your own and be convinced to make them feasible and reachable. Unreachable goals may cause you to become frustrated and feel like your bodyweight loss journey is failing. Set reasonable goals and use apple cider vinegar to assist you in reaching those goals systematically.

Step 9

Maintain a healthy body weight once you achieve your goal weight by avoiding fatty foods and continuing to utilize apple cider vinegar to market healthy weight loss.

Chapter 2
Constituents of ACV

Everybody knows that vinegar continues to be the primary ingredient in a number of common recipes for combating several illnesses. From pickles to salads, we've seen the usage of vinegar as an extremely useful preservative. Moreover, it has additionally been used as a cleaning agent to create mirrors and metallic objects sparkle. It's used as a natural remedy to help people relieve themselves of the possible ailments greatly.

The contents of Apple Cider Vinegar are easy to guess. The name gives everything away. That is a pale, amber-coloured liquid that is produced from cider or apples. To create apple cider vinegar, apples are crushed and squeezed until all of the juices have already been extracted. To the extract, bacteria and yeast are put in to start the fermentation process. This fermentation is recognized as alcoholic fermentation as all of the sugars within the apple extract are changed into alcohol. Vinegar is chemically referred to as acetic acid. Therefore the next step would be to convert the fermented apple extract into vinegar. In this technique, a strain of bacteria that forms acetic acid can be used to convert the alcohol into acetic acid. It is this step that provides apple cider vinegar its trademark sour taste. The initial taste of apple cider vinegar helps it be an excellent ingredient for salad dressings, marinades, vinaigrettes, and also, chutneys.

Types of Apple Cider Vinegar

Vinegar Apple cider vinegar, as we realize now, could be a fermented product produced from apples. You will find two types of apple cider vinegar which are easy to get, and they are:

Raw Apple Cider Vinegar

This is the natural type of apple cider vinegar. It is known because of its strong flavor that works beautifully with different varieties of salads and pickles. The health benefits of raw apple cider vinegar will also be many. You'll be able to recognize raw apple cider vinegar using its color and texture. It is a bright, amber-colored liquid. It includes a cloudy appearance since it contains *"mother of vinegar"* Mother of vinegar is a stringy substance that's naturally formed once the apple extracts are fermented. That is gelatinous in texture and is known to become very best for your health since it contains all of the *'sound bacteria'* as well as the raw *enzymes*.

This sort of apple cider vinegar, although very helpful, is slightly difficult to store. You need to maintain recommended conditions as well as the pH balance from the tonic to make sure that there isn't bacterial growth in it.

Pasteurized Apple Cider Vinegar

Pasteurization is usually a kind of treatment that's directed at foods to make them ideal for consumption. The primary objective of pasteurization would be to destroy certain strains of micro-organisms that may be very bad for health and wellness. In this technique, the apple cider vinegar is subjected to high temperatures where the unwanted microorganisms cannot flourish. Pasteurized apple cider vinegar is clear in its appearance. *It is because the "mother of vinegar" is removed to give it a sparkling clean appearance.* Several health experts argue that technique removes the natural goodness of apple cider vinegar which forms the foundation of all health treatments.

However, storage isn't an issue with pasteurized apple cider vinegar as the probability of bacterial growth is lower. This obvious appearance can be more desirable to consumers, and it is therefore advertised by most manufacturers. The only real common thing between the two types of apple cider vinegar would be that the core element that provides them a characteristic taste and odor may be the acetic acid. However, there are many reasons why you need to select organic apple cider vinegar over the pasteurized variety. We will discuss this at length as you read further, so you can get the exact differentiation and, therefore, understand advantages in the organic variety.

Apple Cider Vinegar and Acid Reflux Disorder

Acid reflux is usually a common digestive disorder. It is known to produce a whole lot of uneasiness and discomfort. Now, *what is acid reflux?*

The entrance to your stomach is controlled with a valve that's called the low esophageal valve, which is a ring of muscles that open and permit the food into the stomach. It also ensures that the food remains there. This makes certain that all of the food plus the digestive enzymes that are produced remain inside the stomach. Sometimes, the valve does not close entirely or might often open to permit the acids to move up the esophagus. This is what we often describe as heartburn or acid reflux disorder.

This condition could be severely painful since it is along with a burning sensation inside the chest. Sometimes this problem is temporary. It could be brought on by prone (after much meal) and, in addition, indulging in midnight snacking. However, it is also an established disease if it occurs a lot more than twice weekly. It's very common in people who are obese or overweight. Additionally, it is quite typical in individuals who are addicted to certain substances of drinks.

This condition can be referred to as *gastroesophageal reflux disease*. Another condition occurring with this disease is *hiatal hernia*. In this problem, the low esophageal valve, along with the stomach more significant than the diaphragm. In cases like this, the diaphragm struggles to keep the acid carefully in your stomach and therefore worsens the problem.

Apple cider vinegar is an extremely common fix for acid reflux disorder and has been used for several years to serve this purpose. What's bizarre or worth some thought is the fact that the proven fact that apple cider vinegar itself is highly acidic. So, how is it feasible it controls acid reflux disorder and its symptoms? Also, acidic foods should never be recommended for those who have acid reflux disorder? So, how could it be that apple cider vinegar cut the set of recommended acid reflux disorder remedies?

Many ideas support this bizarre medical remedy. However, the specific reason for this selection of medication continues to be unknown.

The sole possible explanation for this is the fact that apple cider vinegar contains common enzymes. In the end, apple cider vinegar is a fermented type of apples. Now, apples have already been recommended as the right fix for acid reflux. That is possible because apples have the ability to protect our intestines and therefore reduce the likelihood of acid reflux disorder.

Apple cider vinegar is quite beneficial in reducing the pH degrees of our blood. This, subsequently, helps the intestine fight parasites and fungi that cause acid reflux disorder frequently. Apple cider vinegar also includes proven antimicrobial properties that help maintain intestinal health. When the fitness of the intestine is maintained, the chance of acid reflux disorder is usually reduced to a significant extent. However, this just results in a preventive measure.

Apple Cider Vinegar, alternatively, is useful even though you already are suffering from acid reflux disorder. Based on the Maryland Medical centre, taking two teaspoons of apple cider vinegar with tepid to warm water has the capacity to prevent food poisoning. It may also control the symptoms of acid reflux disorder.

There are a few theories that state the possible ways that apple cider vinegar reacts inside our body to create the required outcome. The first theory is the fact that apple cider vinegar includes a natural acidic property that's valuable in wearing down fats quickly. That is very helpful in accelerating the procedure of digestion. Digestion can be eased to lessen the symptoms of acid reflux disorder.

Other theories claim that the production of acids within the stomach is regulated by using apple cider vinegar.

The acetic acid inside the apple cider vinegar acts as a buffer for the amount of acidity within the stomach. It is because acetic acid isn't as strong as the hydrochloric acid that's stated in the stomach. This acts as a balancing agent and therefore controls the acidity inside our stomach.

While they are only possibilities and ideas, the thing that people know for certain is the fact that apple cider vinegar is highly useful in providing rest from acid reflux disorder. When the product is consumed, especially in its organic form, the vast benefits are numerous. Due to the immediate relief and the future benefits, apple cider vinegar continues to be voted as the utmost reliable natural fix for acid reflux.

Apple Cider Vinegar and Weightloss

Apple cider vinegar is frequently used because of its ability to decrease fats and help us drastically reduce weight. Because of this, apple cider vinegar has found its way into several ancient remedies to keep up physical health.

Today we eat apple cider vinegar through salads as well as tablets to assist weight reduction. With the existing need to appear suitable regularly and to possess the most popular hour-glass figure, several celebrities and health experts have considered apple cider vinegar to be the best natural fat loss remedy. This ingredient, when made an integral part of our standard diet, has the capacity to decrease weight, make you feel more energetic, and improve our overall wellness. The very best part is definitely that we now have no severe unwanted effects.

This product is natural and safe and also the best weight-loss solution open to us today.

Ancient recipes claim that apple cider vinegar can reduce appetite and food craving when consumed in the right quantities. Metabolism can be stimulated whenever you consume apple cider vinegar. That is probably one of the most crucial requirements if you are currently around the route to dropping weight.

Weight loss can be significantly accelerated by apple cider vinegar since it can regulate the blood sugar inside our body. This can help suppress hunger and, for that reason, control your daily diet effectively.

Studies have already been conducted to comprehend the partnership between weight reduction and apple cider vinegar consumption. In '09 2009, a report carried out in Japan showed a substantial influence on obese individuals when apple cider vinegar was administered to them frequently. These individuals received just 30ml of vinegar every day. This caused a substantial reduction in their weight as well as their appetite. This study revealed that vinegar intake includes a lot of results on surplus fat mass maintenance and in addition, body weight regulation. It is because of acetic acid that's beneficial in reducing the accumulation of fat in the torso.

Including apple cider vinegar in what you eat is usually recommended if you're looking at an all-natural and effective fat loss routine. Apple cider vinegar has the capacity to increase your metabolism and, hence, increase your chances of slimming down. Studies linked to apple cider vinegar and weight-loss also claim that it is highly beneficial in maintaining the sugar balance in the torso. The glycemic index of particular foods is usually reduced when apple cider vinegar is consumed. This property helps spike weight reduction.

Apple cider vinegar also offers the capability to control conditions like *candida*. That is a fungal infection that triggers cravings for sugars and carbohydrates. This plays a part in weight gain, which is considerably controlled through the use of apple cider vinegar, which has popular anti-fungal properties.

The intake of apple cider vinegar has another vital result that is detoxification. The apple cider vinegar detox is among the most crucial fitness remedies nowadays. Since apple cider vinegar is incredibly acidic in nature, it has the capacity to boost digestion. Furthermore, These enzymes have become valuable and form the foundation of all health advantages of apple vinegar cider. The procedure version is, without a doubt very clear and nicer looking. Nevertheless, the nutritional benefits, along with other health benefits of the type of apple vinegar cider, are fewer.

Apple Cider Vinegar for the Hair

Apple Cider Vinegar is a superb treatment for the hair. Though it may appear just like a rather unconventional method, Apple Cider Vinegar, when blended with other 100% natural ingredients like *Greek Yogurt and Honey*, can transform the looks of the hair. Here are some ways that you should use Apple Cider Vinegar for the hair.

1. ***As a Hair Conditioner:*** If you're fighting frizzy and unmanageable hair, the thing you need is an excellent conditioner. Apple Cider Vinegar ought to be rubbed

softly into the scalp and along the space of your respective hair having a dash of baking soda. This combination nourishes and conditions hair leaving it soft, smooth, and supple.

2. **Increasing Porosity with the Hair:** Our hair maintains its natural sheen due to its capability to hold moisture within it. This characteristic on the hair is recognized as porosity. When hair does not absorb moisture and keep it locked within itself, it causes an extremely brittle hair shaft. Since this hair becomes lifeless, which is susceptible to breakage. Using Apple Cider Vinegar within the hair can improve porosity. It is because the acidity of Apple Cider Vinegar seals the cuticle from the hair and therefore allows it to retain moisture.

3. **Manage Tangles:** Hair breaks and falls at a significant rate when it's difficult to comb hair very quickly. One of the primary contributors to hair breakage is hair tangles. Using Apple Cider Vinegar along the distance in the hair keeps it well moisturized since the top of hair also flattens out, rendering it simple to detangle the hair. We will

observe that with frequent use, it gets easier to glide the comb down with the hair.

4. **<u>Treat Hair Loss</u>:** When hair becomes more manageable and much more conditioned, it is less susceptible to breakage and damage. Most hair loss is due to breakage while combing the hair. Using Apple Cider Vinegar reduces the probability of hair loss because of tangled hair; moreover, the acidic houses Apple Cider Vinegar also cleans from the oil glands present below the hair follicle. This stimulates hair regrowth and makes your locks longer and thicker.

5. **<u>Cleansing on the Scalp</u>:** Most of us disregard the need for our scalp as part of our hair treatment regimen. However, besides regular shampooing and washing our hair requires additional care to make sure that the scalp is clear of dry skin and dandruff. It is smart to apply an assortment of Apple Cider Vinegar and baking soda for the scalp for an intensive cleansing routine. Many people have found this combination so useful which they entirely replaced shampoos as well as other chemical-based products with this natural and economical option.

6. **Clarifying Treatment**: Whenever we use chemically treated hair products, there's always some residue actually after thorough washing. Over a period, these chemicals build-up inside the scalp and make our hair weak and brittle. It's essential to make sure that the chemical build-up is removed frequently. Apple Cider Vinegar is an ideal product for this function. It is because it is strong enough to eliminate the chemical but can be mild enough to make sure that the scalp isn't stripped of its oils.

7. **PH Balance:** To be able to grow our hair properly takes a recommended pH level, which is based on the number of 4.5 to 5.5. This implies that our hair is mildly acidic in nature, and it needs a product that may maintain this acidity. The glad tidings are that Apple Cider Vinegar comes with an acidity that's nearly the same as our hair. So that it is recommended which you rinse hair with Apple Cider Vinegar every time you shampoo it to make sure that the pH level is retained.

8. **Controlling Frizz:** Frizzy hair always looks unkempt and can be challenging to control and often becomes brittle if left untreated. Apple Cider Vinegar, along with baking soda, is an ideal frizz control treatment. This technique ensures that the procedure reaches every strand of the hair. Because of this, all of the strays are controlled, and every strand of hair becomes shinier and better to maintain. Naturally, it is visually pleasing as the hair appears like it is in place and not simply one big unmanageable bunch.

9. **Treatment of Itchy and Dry Scalp:** Apple Cider Vinegar is well known for its capability to fight bacteria and fungus. Often infections like certain strains of bacteria or viruses make the scalp itchy, dry, and flaky. In a few severe conditions, scabs are produced on the top of the scalp. When these fall or are plucked, they release pus that blocks the oil glands present below the hair follicle. Because of this, the hair will not have the nourishment that it needs. Consequently, it becomes weak and dull.

10. **Prevention of Split Ends:** Split Ends gives our hair the looks to be very unmanageable and dull. Additionally, it is thought that split ends prevent hair regrowth and also

result in lifeless hair. Regularly rinsing beautiful hair with Apple Cider Vinegar helps control this problem. Moreover, flowing hair also gets a lovely bounce, since hair loss also reduces, the quantity increases automatically.

Apple Cider Vinegar is, without a doubt, one of the better options for excellent natural hair care treatment. It is available easily, can be inexpensive and can be very easy to use. It is no wonder which it finds a location generally in most natural remedies. You can even make ready your own Apple Cider Vinegar in the home.

All you have to accomplish is mix a part of warm water to 1 portion of Apple Cider Vinegar. Ensure that the water you are employing is filtered. Following the standard shampooing regimen, all you have to do is certainly apply this homemade rinse. In the event you think hair needs more conditioning, you might leave it on your hair for two minutes before you rinse off with water. It is strongly recommended that you utilize this hair care product at least one time week for optimum results.

Apple Cider Vinegar for Skin

Many adolescents and adults have a problem with the issue of acne. Only a few understand that Apple Cider Vinegar is a beneficial product to help look after the skin and remove pimples forever significantly. Of all house care remedies which are recommended it's been observed that Apple Cider Vinegar may be the most reliable one. The question is how Apple Cider Vinegar aids the betterment of skin compared to other products?

Apple Cider Vinegar that is created from organic apples and has been left unfiltered includes a substance referred to as the mother of vinegar. It is with this cloudy substance that several enzymes and minerals that are advantageous to your skin are found. Therefore it will always be recommended you shake your bottle of Apple Cider Vinegar well each time you utilize it so that these enzymes are released into the liquid.

Apple Cider Vinegar gets the same constituents as apples. One particular component is normally malic acid which contributes largely to your skincare using Apple Cider

Vinegar. This component gives Apple Cider Vinegar its antibacterial, anti-fungal feature. This can help it prevent acne and skin infections and also, combat common dermatological problems. Probably one of the most contributing factors for acne is the production of excessive oil within the glands present at the bottom of the skin we have. Apple Cider Vinegar works by removing this excess oil to make sure that these glands aren't infected to produce outbursts and acne. The maintenance of the pH balance of the skin is another essential function of Apple Cider Vinegar. It means that the oil secretion in your skin is usually normalized to make sure that it doesn't become too dry or too oily.

Apple Cider Vinegar also acts as an excellent exfoliating agent. You'll want to be pointed out that most commercial skincare products which can be priced high advertise the current presence of alpha-hydroxy acids within their preparation. However, Apple Cider Vinegar forms a cheaper and far more effective option for the products. The role of alpha-hydroxy acids is usually to eliminate the layer of dead skin cells, to supply a wholesome complexion. Also, the layer of skin beneath the dead skin is a fresher and healthier one which plays a part in the youthful glow that Apple Cider Vinegar promises.

Age spots are another common dermatological problem that lots of women grapple with. It's been discovered that mixing Apple Cider Vinegar with fresh orange juice as well as onion juice provides desirable results. All you have to do is to apply this mixture over these spots many times per day. If your skin layer is usually sensitive, this application may sting slightly. However, you don't have to panic since it is not the medial side effect.

Apple Cider Vinegar is among the only natural basic products that are effective in treating warts. A little ball of cotton wool soaked in Apple Cider Vinegar and pressed contrary to the wart using a tape or band-aid may be the most reliable remedy. You may keep this application on all day long, or you might just use overnight. It's been observed that warts get rid of within weekly. You have to understand that the wart will turn completely black before it falls off. If you continue to make use of Apple Cider

Vinegar even following warts, possess gone, you will be confident that they could not appear again.

Apple Cider Vinegar, when consumed internally, promotes healthy skin. This is because it detoxifies your body and treats any condition linked to digestion. Apple Cider Vinegar promotes better functioning of your liver. The primary function of a healthy liver can be to eliminate toxins from your body. Usually, the liver is overworked due to poor digestion. It has an effect on your skin which may be the first reflection of any toxic overload in the torso.

For individuals who only have confidence in the topical application of Apple Cider Vinegar, you can create your own apple vinegar face wash at home. All you have to do is certainly mix Apple Cider Vinegar with water in a 1:3 ratio. If you are accustomed to using Apple Cider Vinegar, you may make this face wash more concentrated and talk about the ratio to at least one 1:1.

To make certain that the skin isn't oversensitive to Apple Cider Vinegar, a patch test is definitely recommended.

Apply a little to your elbow or any hidden section of that person. Allow this mixture to take a seat on your skin layer for one hour to check out any adverse reaction. When there is a problem, you might work with Apple Cider Vinegar in a much-diluted form. Once you've become comfortable using Apple Cider Vinegar as a face-wash, you can use it regularly in your beauty regimen. In the first place wash that spot with normal lukewarm water, clean that person with a cotton ball dipped in Apple Cider Vinegar. Encompass the entire region together with your neck. Ensure that all of the strokes you utilize are upward and gentle.

You should use Apple Cider Vinegar to generate deep core treatment packs that may remove any dirt and grime on your face. An assortment of Apple Cider Vinegar, Honey and fullers earth clay could be applied on your skin and left for 10 to quarter-hour. Whenever you wash it off, you will observe that your skin layer is supple and soft.

Many people have found beneficial skin remedies simply by replacing their usual toner with Apple Cider Vinegar.

You can just to use an assortment of Apple Cider Vinegar and water around your skin layer. This means that your complexion is clear, and all of the freckles and age spots diminish. Also, it prevents the accumulation of cellulite on your face.

Apple Cider Vinegar can be known for fighting signs of aging. It is because it contains a great deal of Sulfur- which helps in tightening your skin and in addition, reducing the probability of fine lines and wrinkles. It is strongly recommended that you apply Apple Cider Vinegar on the face each night and wash it off with water the following day.

Apple Cider Vinegar can be a robust astringent. It is therefore valuable against any inflammation that could be located on the skin. Additionally, it is effective against sunburns. All you need to do is apply a modest amount of Apple Cider Vinegar in the affected area for immediate results.

The thumb rule to utilize Apple Cider Vinegar is that you need to dilute it when you feel a sting on the skin. This pinch or sting is just caused because your skin layer is sensitive and isn't any side-effect on using Apple Cider Vinegar.

Health Benefits of Organic ACV

Proponents declare that apple cider vinegar may increase your health in many ways. Science backs up a few of these claims. As you read further, you would learn the various way with which Apple Cider Vinegar can be useful for numerous health condition healing, including the recipes needed and method of use.

Blood Sugar

The acetic acid in Vinegar seems to block enzymes that assist you to digest starch, producing a smaller glucose level response after starchy meals such as pasta or bread. A 2017 overview of studies published in Diabetes Research & Clinical Practice suggested that the increased intake of Vinegar with meals can decrease fluctuations in insulin and blood sugar levels after meals.

To include apple cider vinegar in meals, make an effort adding a splash to salads, marinades, vinaigrettes, and sauces. If you have *diabetes or prediabetes*, make sure to check with your doctor if you're considering using amounts larger than those generally within cooking. Vinegar can interact with diabetes medication, and it must not be used by people who have specific health issues, like gastroparesis.

Weight Loss

Proponents declare that consuming Vinegar before or with meals may have a satiating effect. A 12-week study from Japan conducted reported that people who had consumed as much as 30 millilitres (roughly 6 teaspoons) of Vinegar each day experienced a modest one-to-two pound decrease in body weight. Body mass index (BMI), waist circumference, triglycerides, and visceral fat were also slightly reduced.

People tend to consume higher than normal levels of apple cider vinegar when working with it for weight loss purposes, with some even taking it in tablet form.

How to use Apple Cider Vinegar in Your Daily Diet.

There are many methods for you to add apple cider vinegar to your daily diet that tastes great and packs a nutritional punch. Here are some of the favourites;

Salad Dressing

Raise your salad by substituting your usual balsamic for apple cider vinegar. Just mix it with healthy oils, herbs, and spices. That is a terrific way to sneak in a few extra health advantages. You can even buy premade dressings that use ACV among the main ingredients.

Probiotic Tonic

Make an effort to make your tonic by mixing apple cider vinegar with fruit than one sweet. Allow it to sit for a couple of days in the refrigerator. Pop in several fresh berries for added color and flavor for a great probiotic drink!

Marinade

Another creative way to include apple cider vinegar into your daily diet is by using it as a tenderizer if you are cooking meat or poultry. Mix it with herbs and spices to produce your marinade recipe.

Cocktails or drinks

Having a celebration? Make an effort adding ACV for your spiked cider or Bloody Mary mix recipes. Still uncertain about the taste? You can even obtain apple cider vinegar in capsule or pill form and take it this way. **Warning:** The capsules will still smell like apple cider vinegar.

Other Uses of ACV

Over time, apple cider vinegar continues to be used as a home remedy for a lot of health insurance and beauty issues. While there is not strong science to back these claims, there exists some anecdotal evidence to affirm its potential.

Dandruff

To handle dandruff, some individuals discover that lightly spritzing an apple cider vinegar and water solution onto the scalp combats persistent flakes, itchiness, and irritation. Vinegar's acetic acid may alter the scalp's pH, rendering it harder for yeast - *one of the primary contributors to dandruff to flourish*. There are also suggestions that it could treat a kind of eczema referred to as seborrheic dermatitis.

A 2017 study published within the Galen Medical Journal suggested the topical application of the flowering herb *Althaea officinalis* coupled with the Vinegar could resolve seborrheic dermatitis.

Although apple cider vinegar may also be recommended being a hair rinse to eliminate shampoo build-up and clarify dull hair, the answer must be diluted to avoid stinging the eyes.

Dry Scalp Sunburn along with other Skin Injuries

While the more common recommendation for any mild sunburn is a cold water compress, refreshing bath, aloe gel, or moisturizer, some individuals sweat by apple cider vinegar. It could be added to an excellent bath or blended with cold water and lightly spritzed on affected areas (preventing the face) to alleviate discomfort and pain.

There is certainly little evidence that apple cider vinegar might help heal or relieve sunburn pain much better than no treatment. It can, however, have an excellent antibacterial effect that might help prevent skin infections due to sunburn as well as other skin injuries.

Apple cider vinegar shouldn't be employed full-strength or in substantial concentrations to your skin, as the acidity can further injure your skin. In addition, it shouldn't be utilized for much more severe burns. Make sure to consult your doctor for assistance in determining the severe nature of the sunburn.

When you have mosquito bites, poison ivy, or jellyfish stings, a weak apple cider vinegar solution dabbed onto bites and stings can help itching and irritation.

Acne and other Chronic Skin Disorders

Apple cider vinegar can help to dry pimples whenever a solution is dabbed onto pimples. It ought to be diluted before putting it on to the facial skin as it could cause skin injury or chemical burns if it's not diluted enough.

The concentration of acetic acid in apple cider vinegar varies widely and isn't standardized, rendering it difficult to gauge just how much to dilute it to be safe as a skin toner or for various other purposes.

Although the data supporting the usage of apple cider vinegar in treating acne is not conclusive due to a few shortcomings, research has suggested that it could help diminish the looks of varicose veins when applied topically.

Sore Throat

A time-honored throat elixir, apple cider vinegar drinks, and gargles are thought to alleviate the pain of any sore throat (*pharyngitis*). Although there are various recipes and protocols, a simple drink recipe demands a teaspoon of apple cider vinegar, a teaspoon of honey, and a little pinch of cayenne pepper stirred inside a cup of tepid to warm water.

Although proponents declare that apple cider vinegar has germ-fighting properties, and capsaicin in chile peppers alleviates pain, there hasn't been any research on apple cider vinegar's capability to fight sore throats. Moreover, there may be evidence that treating a sore throat with Vinegar could cause considerably more harm than sound.

If not adequately diluted, Vinegar can corrode esophageal tissues, causing persistent throat pain and dysphagia (difficulty swallowing). It is unclear at what concentration apple cider vinegar would be safe for use in treating pharyngitis, particularly in children.

Deodorant for Smelly Feet

To keep smelly feet in order, proponents claim apple cider vinegar can help to balance the skin's pH and fight the bacteria that trigger foot odor. Typically, a little bit of apple cider vinegar is mixed into water. Baby wipes, cotton balls or pads, small towels, or cotton rags could be dipped into the solution, wrung out, and utilized to wipe underneath of your toes. Wipes could be made ahead and stored within an airtight container.

Although a vinegar scent will be noticed, it often dissipates once the vinegar solution has dried. Avoid wearing shoes created from materials like leather that may be damaged with the acidity. *An apple cider vinegar solution may also help neutralize odor-causing armpit bacteria.* Typically, cotton pads, towelettes, or cotton rags are lightly spritzed with a weak solution and swiped onto the armpits. The vinegar smell should dissipate since it dries. It's wise to check the apple cider vinegar solution within a smaller region first, also to stay away from it if you are wearing delicate fibers, like silk.

Is Apple Cider Vinegar Safe?

It is time to talk about Apple Cider Vinegar's safety. Generally, eating it in smaller amounts is safe. However, many doctors claim that you do not consume a lot more than 8 ounces each day because it continues to be linked to several unwanted effects, like low potassium levels, which may cause muscle cramps or weakness and when it gets extreme could be dangerous. Also, when you have diabetes, speak to your doctor since it can lower blood sugar levels. When you have any kind of chronic health, it is smart to check with your doctor before making a decision to supplement with it. Additionally, it is recommended you don't drink it straight since it is quite acidic and may consequently harm your esophagus and perhaps contribute to tooth and tooth enamel decay. (In addition, it tastes pretty terrible doing this, TBH.)

Apple cider vinegar is a liquid produced through the fermentation of apple cider. In this procedure, the sugar in apples is fermented by yeast and/or bacteria put into the cider, which in turn converts it into alcohol and, finally, into Vinegar. Like other styles of Vinegar, the main element component in apple cider vinegar is acetic acid. Apple cider vinegar also includes other substances like lactic, citric, and malic acids, and bacteria.

For years, apple cider vinegar has been used as a home remedy to take care of many health ailments as a disinfectant and natural preservative.

Side Effects of ACV

Apple cider vinegar is a favorite household ingredient, which might cause you to think that it's completely safe.

While there could be no cause for alarm if you're generally healthy, there are a few potential effects to understand, especially if the concentration is too intense or is definitely in contact with the body for too much time.

Apple cider vinegar, for example, could cause chemical burns. There were case reports of chemical burns after apple cider vinegar was used for warts and a condition of the skin referred to as *Molluscum contagiosum*.

Although apple cider vinegar is widely touted like a do-it-yourself solution to whiten teeth or freshen breath, exposing your teeth to the acidity may erode tooth enamel and result in cavities.

When taken internally, ACV may bring about decreased potassium amounts, hypoglycemia, throat irritation, and allergies. It is an acid (a pH lower than 7 is an acid, and many apple cider vinegar products have a pH of 2 to 3). It can cause burns and injury to the digestive tract (including the throat, esophagus, and stomach), especially when taken undiluted or in large amounts.

Apple cider vinegar may interact with certain medications, including laxatives, diuretics, blood thinners, and cardiovascular disease and diabetes medications. Apple cider vinegar shouldn't be utilized as a nose spray, sinus wash, or in a neti pot, and it shouldn't be put into eye drops. Vinegar won't assist in the treatment of lice.

Dosage and Preparation

Apple cider vinegar can be obtained being a liquid and in supplement capsules. There is absolutely no standard dose for ACV supplements, so follow the package directions and seek advice from your doctor.

When working with Vinegar, most suggested uses involve diluting apple cider vinegar before putting it on to your body. However, the safety of different vinegar-to-water ratios isn't known. A 1:10 ratio has been suggested when putting it right to the skin. However, it ought to be weaker in concentration (or prevented entirely) on weak or delicate skin.

Although a teaspoon to some tablespoon mixed into 8 ounces of water is often suggested as an acceptable amount for internal use, the safety of varied doses isn't known.

You can test to use it when highly diluted; however, the amount of acetic acid in commercial apple cider vinegar varies (unlike white Vinegar, that is 5% acetic acid), rendering it impossible to be certain from the actual strength.

What to Watch out For:

Apple cider vinegar can be found filtered or unfiltered. Filtered apple cider is a distinct light brown color. Unfiltered and unpasteurized ACV (such as *Bragg's apple cider vinegar*) has dark, cloudy sediment in the bottom in the bottle. Referred to as *"mother of vinegar"* or just *"the mother,"* this sediment consists mainly of acetic acid bacteria. Apple cider vinegar can be available in tablet form.

When buying apple cider vinegar in supplement form, browse the product label to make sure that apple cider vinegar is listed inside the ingredients instead of acetic acid (white vinegar).

Recipes

A splash of apple cider vinegar can brighten many dishes (not only salads) and add excellent flavor to your cooking. Check it out in these recipes:

- Low-carb pomegranate salad with cider walnut vinaigrette.
- Smoky baked bean medley.
- Pulled pork barbecue sauce.
- Vegan goddess dressing.

Numerous anecdotal uses plus some preliminary evidence are suggesting that it could help certain conditions. However, you might realize that you reap the benefits of its homes, large-scale clinical trials are needed before it could be recommended as a cure for any health.

If you're considering using apple cider vinegar for just about any health purpose, make sure to consult with your doctor to see if it's best for you, as opposed to self-treating and avoiding or delaying standard treatment. Individuals with certain conditions (like ulcers, hiatal hernia, Barrett's esophagus, or low potassium) might need to avoid apple cider vinegar entirely.

Methods for Safe Use of ACV

Regularly consuming significant levels of undiluted Vinegar can result in side effects.

One is much more likely to experience adverse effects if they regularly consume large quantities of undiluted Vinegar or leave it on the skin for very long periods.

To lower the chance of unwanted side effects, try:

- reducing the amount of Vinegar consumed,
- reducing the quantity of time that Vinegar touches your skin diluting the Vinegar with water or using it as an ingredient limiting connection with your teeth by drinking the Vinegar via a straw.

A 2016 review discovered that people might be able to achieve lots of potential health advantages by drinking around 15 milliliters of Vinegar each day or any quantity that contains around 750 milligrams of acetic acid.

However, due to having less research into unwanted effects and long-term safety, further moderation could be the very best approach. People who have digestive issues, low potassium levels, or diabetes should think about speaking to a health care provider before consuming apple cider vinegar. Anyone who experiences severe unwanted effects should consult with a medical professional, consuming apple cider vinegar has turned into a popular health trend.

Some evidence shows that Vinegar can help with a variety of medical issues. However, scientists have to carry out even more research to verify and understand these findings. Apple cider vinegar could cause unwanted effects; for instance, applying undiluted Vinegar to your skin for very long periods can result in burns and irritation. Regularly consuming significant levels of the Vinegar, especially within an undiluted kind, could cause digestive issues, damage one's teeth, and affect potassium levels. Anyone who experiences severe unwanted effects after using apple cider vinegar should seek health care.

Debunking great medical things about apple cider vinegar
The Internet could have you think apple cider vinegar may be the new pixie dust because of its health advantages. It's tempting to trust the web claims about apple cider vinegar

(ACV). They sound so fantastic that even doctors can fall victim to them if not carefully handled or administered.

Chapter 3
Household Benefits of Apple Cider Vinegar

Apple Cider vinegar is among the most effective cleansing agents within nature. It's the strong acidic property of the substance that means it is extremely useful in household applications. Many homes choose the usage of apple cider vinegar over chemically available products as this is the healthiest as well as the most obvious decision for those who are worried about the wellbeing of their family. The uses of Apple Cider Vinegar in a household include the following as:

Being a cleansing agent

Apple Cider Vinegar is ideal for cleaning household appliances. All you have to do is mix some of apple cider vinegar with water and use it on the region of your home or the appliance that you would like to completely clean. The acidic property of Apple Cider Vinegar means that any scum or soap residue that is seen in appliances and regions of the house like the bathroom or the kitchen is removed very quickly. When the mildew, grime or scum in your shower area, the bathtub or even the tiles of your kitchen is bothering you, all you need to do is spray a generous amount of Apple Cider Vinegar and wipe it off after a while.

Remove oil from pots and pans

The most common problem that we face with pots and pans is the accumulation of oil and even food stains over a period. This makes the utensils quite undesirable to look at. In such cases, all you need to do is apply a generous amount of Apple Cider Vinegar on the vessel. Following this, you must just rinse the utensils in hot water to make sure that all the stains are gone.

Cleaning Windows

If you dread cleaning your windows because it is a time-consuming process, it is recommended that you give Apple Cider Vinegar a shot. All you need to do is spray Apple Cider Vinegar on the window panes and wipe them completely clean. The stains, the grime and the dust, are removed by the acidic nature of Apple Cider Vinegar, making your job a lot easier.

Removing stains from your carpet

If you have pets at home, then the most common problem that you will face is that of stubborn stains of your carpet. Even marks like wine spills or even sauce stains can be extremely hard to get rid of. In such cases, using Apple Cider Vinegar can be of great help. All you need to do is mix equal portions of Apple Cider Vinegar and water. Run this mixture over the stain several times. When you are sure that the stain is gone completely, all you have to accomplish is blot the surplus liquid. Once your carpet is dry, the stain will vanish entirely.

Removing lime build-up

By using hard water comes perhaps one of the most challenging household problems- Lime build-up. The areas which might be most affected will be the shower enclosures plus the tiles of your bathrooms. The deposits leave the tiles looking old and lifeless. If you're after a quick fix for this issue, I recommend Apple Cider Vinegar as a highly effective measure.

Deodorizing your house

Apple Cider Vinegar pays in removing any undesirable smell from your household. If you find that a particular room in your house has a strong cigarette smell or any other strong odour, all you need to do is place a jar of apple cider vinegar in the room somewhere. Sometimes, even the garbage disposal develops a peculiar odour that can make its way to any corner of your home. In such cases, all you need to do is pour a cup of Apple Cider Vinegar along with ice cubes into the garbage disposal.

Keeping ants away

If your home is attacked and invaded by ants frequently, Apple Cider Vinegar might be the solution that you are looking for. All you need to do is spray a mixture of vinegar with an equal proportion of water. Make sure you cover/close all the entry points of these pests into your home. This includes the window sills, the door and any small hole of a gap that the ants can make their way into your house through, to enhance the effectiveness.

Prevent fading of clothes

If you are worried about your clothes fading away in the sun, you can use Apple Cider Vinegar as a useful preventive measure. All you need to do is soak your clothes in water containing Apple Cider Vinegar before washing them. This way, even though they may be dried in sunlight, clothes will stay bright and can look new at all times.

Prevent the formation of ice in your windshield

In case you are sick of getting up every morning and spending lots of time defrosting your window shield, you might like to dig out the jar of Apple Cider Vinegar in your closet. *To prevent the deposit of ice, all you need to do is pour two cups of Apple Cider Vinegar over the windshield and then rinse it off with a little water.*

Removing Wall Paper

If you are considering getting rid of the wallpaper in your home, you need not worry. It is not a very difficult process if you have Apple Cider Vinegar at home. All you need to do is make a mixture of hot water and apple cider vinegar in equal parts. Now rub this over the wallpaper that you want to remove. When the mixture is soaked in completely, the wallpaper will begin to peel off on its own.

Flowers and Grass

When you have an unwanted weed growing in your bed of flowers and grass, all you have to accomplish is pour Apple Cider Vinegar inside the affected area to prevent further weed growth.

Apple Cider Vinegar has other uses in children. The end result is that this strong acidic property of Apple Cider Vinegar helps it be an extremely powerful cleansing agent. In addition, it helps it be a disinfectant and a trusted deodorizer. You can prefer to get Apple Cider Vinegar from the store or can make it in the home to discover the best results.

Chapter 4
Apple Cider Vinegar for Healing Numerous Health Conditions

"An apple each day keeps the doctor away" is a familiar saying to millions. It has good sense. The apple is among God's wonderful health-giving foods. Apples certainly are a fruitful way to get potassium, which is usually to the soft tissues of your body as calcium would be to the bones and harder tissues. Potassium may be the mineral of youthfulness; it's the *"artery softener,"* keeping the arteries of your body flexible and resilient.

It is a fighter of dangerous bacteria and viruses. Yes, whenever you state, *"An apple per day keeps the doctor away," you are saying something good*, down-to-earth old-fashioned natural medicine for vibrant, life-long health! The apple has stood the test of time. It is among the oldest known fruits that humans consume. The Garden of Eden, the apple, has played an essential part in our destiny. People have been consuming apples for a large number of years. Apple eaters possess a particular healthfulness that non-apple eaters never achieve. Apples are delicious fruits that many people enjoy eating; potassium may be the key mineral within the constellation of nutrients; it's so vital that without it, there will be no life! Most humans are deficient in potassium, and it reflects within their cell tissues and throughout their overall body. Check around you, how many people would you see which have the super glow of health?

There is absolutely no wealth higher than the fitness of the body.

Problems with Potassium Deficiency

Millions surviving in today's civilization and feeding on its commercialized processed food items have got a potassium deficiency. The skin and muscle tone are bad. The flesh will not cling firmly towards the body's bony framework. Lines and wrinkles fill the facial skin and neck. One sign is flabby, excess skin hanging on the eyes. When the potassium deficiency continues, the prolapsing eyelids progress. Soon, people are searching for little slits rather than wide-open eyes. *Thousands have considered eyelid surgery to improve droopy eyelids, also known as hooded eyelids*, that roll down and rest on the eyelashes causing eyestrain, headaches, etc. If an eye doctor suggests corrective surgery because of this, the insurance provider usually honors the claim. It's an in/out local procedure.

It's best; the surgeon is board certified. People wrongly blame how old they are for his or her droopy eyelids, skin changes, and insufficient muscle tone. Nevertheless, you'll want potassium to create and keep maintaining youthful, healthy tissues! *If you don't get the needed amount of potassium daily, you will soon acquire an old-age appearance.* This premature aging is generally because of potassium deficiency and unhealthy living! It's the same within your flower and vegetable garden. Potassium is essential for the production from the substances that provide rigidity to plant stems and increase their resistance to the countless diseases that attack plants. Potassium can be a powerful element that changes seeds into plants and beautiful flowers by progressive development. If plants become deficient in potassium, they stop their growth. In the event the potassium deficiency isn't corrected, the plant slowly starts to wither, turns yellow and dies! The same will apply to animals and humans having a potassium deficiency. There's a slow degeneration resulting in death in the cells, then the loss of life.

Apple Cider Vinegar for Body Cleansing

If time changes and you are feeling bad and don't appear to possess the Human Go Power and Vital Force to accomplish the things in life that are essential! It's time for you to flush out the power depleting, problem causing toxic wastes which are clogging your system and organs of elimination! Waste material divided by this ACV procedure is flushed out. Remember, your essential organs of elimination will be the colon, the lungs, your skin as well as the kidneys. They may be your faithful servants! They work hard 24 hours per day to detox and flush out toxic wastes. Often these eliminative organs need help, and then the ACV drink comes to their aid! Follow the ACV daily program as you would learn as you read further.

Furthermore, *mix 1 tsp of ACV to 6 ounces of salt-free tomato or fresh vegetable juice (carrot and greens) and drink between meals, daily.*

Make sure to execute a cleansing, fast one day weekly and faithfully follow *the lifestyle,* that would be explained further in this chapter.

Apple Cider Vinegar Relieves Headaches

People blame their headaches on a variety of organs of their body. Most headaches are blamed to the eyes, the nerves, the liver, the sinuses, the stomach, the bowel, kidneys, or allergies. Headaches could be placed into two different classifications: One kind of chronic headache could be connected with toxic build-up and illness. A headache can be an alarm telling the individual that deep down within their body; destruction is certainly going on. *Pain and headaches are Mother Nature's great red flashing warning signal to consider fast action!* There could be trouble anywhere through the entire body. Maybe it's inside the liver, gallbladder, kidneys, bowel, or the body's organs.

It might be linked to or due to sensitive sinus, allergy or mucus problems, etc. Avoid these headache trigger foods:

- ✓ Additive and chemical-laced foods
- ✓ Caffeine-containing foods
- ✓ Salty, sugary or wheat-based foods
- ✓ Condiments, sulfites, MSG
- ✓ Dairy foods, especially cheese
- ✓ Alcohol, beer, wine.

The second kind of headache is emotional! This is due to nervousness, anxiety, stress, strain, tension, or any personal or emotional upsets. Your lifestyle with others can toss you into many upsetting emotional problems because they can arouse emotions of fear, jealousy, envy, hate, greed, self-pity, or self-indulgence. When emotions reach a boiling stage, you can end up getting a dull, throbbing headache. The worst headache maybe the migraine, which in turn causes the sufferer to feel like their head is splitting.

We've discovered within our long time of research on all sorts of headaches that whenever your body triggers a headache, the urine is alkaline as opposed to the normal acid. The kidneys are disturbed from the emotions, and this means the body is off-balance. The quickly working malic acid of ACV might help relieve headaches by aiding the kidneys to bring back urine on track (average 6.4 pH) acidity. Vaporized ACV may also help relieve headaches.

Inside a vaporizer or small pan, put 2 Tbsps of ACV and 2 cups of purified water. Bring mixture to boil. As vapor begins to go up, turn the heat off, put towel overhead, and lean over steam, taking five deep, slow breaths of ACV steam vapors.

Also, try hot and cold vinegar compresses to forehead & entire neck area, then do some shoulder/neck rolls, and massage head and shoulders, and when needed, visit your Chiropractor.

*For pain, use **Bromelain 500 mg** - it acts like aspirin with no toxic stomach upset. Many chronic headache sufferers have told us they get blessed relief with this technique.*

By doing these exact things and following this healthy lifestyle, you should have no dependence on commercial headache remedies and pain killers!

ACV Improves Weight Loss Greatly

Whether it's a New Year's resolution, the next wedding, preparation for bikini season, or among so multiple reasons millions choose to start weight loss programs, people spend vast amounts of dollars each year to lose excess weight. Yet lots of the weight loss supplements, portions, and plans neglect to deliver, departing those who paid sense duped, but still wanting to drop those annoying pounds. *The program with the best achievement rate for slimming down and maintaining weight reduction involves an excellent, clean exercise and diet routine,* and apple cider vinegar would help too!

Including ACV inside your weight-loss plan is simple to accomplish and effective.

To produce a daily dose, combine:
- ✓ 1 cup of water
- ✓ 1 tablespoon of ACV
- ✓ 1 tablespoon of lemon juice

Drink the concoction as much as five occasions daily ahead of meals to take pleasure from the many health advantages that can assist in weight loss.

Many people cite the next four obstacles in achieving and maintaining weight loss:

i. Not having the ability to control hunger/cravings
ii. Having an insatiable appetite
iii. Insufficient vigor
iv. A slow metabolism

The naturally occurring elements in ACV would help you overcome every one of those challenges. As you read further, you would get more on how best to use ACV for weight-loss accomplishment.

Fast Body Metabolism

Natural metabolism is a thing that just *"skinny"* people have, right? **Wrong!**

Genetics do play an essential role in metabolism, but anybody can improve his or her metabolic rate naturally. Try out these invigorating ACV recipes.

To produce a drink, combine:

- ✓ 1 cup of green tea extract
- ✓ 2 tablespoons of ACV
- ✓ 1 tablespoon of lemon juice
- ✓ 1 teaspoon of ground cayenne pepper.

To utilize, drink this metabolism-boosting tonic thirty minutes before each meal.

The mix of caffeinated green tea extract, internal-temperature-raising cayenne pepper, and multiple minerals and vitamins in lemon juice and ACV promotes proper metabolic functioning, improves the reduction of fat, and increases energy.

Additionally, try these simple changes in lifestyle to improve your metabolic rates in just a matter of weeks:

Implement a strength-training routine made to increase fat-burning muscle tissue. Eat smaller sized meals more frequently during the day, and also include 30-minute bouts of cardio exercise 4-6 days weekly.

Suppress Your Appetite

Ever been on a diet, peering into the refrigerator, searching for something to prevent your stomach from growling?

Even though you've had the opportunity to adhere to your diet, consume clean foods, and drink plenty of water, you'll still end up hungry and using a seemingly insatiable appetite that's sure to result in diet derailment very quickly. Rather than surrendering to temptation or endure the feelings of starvation and deprivation, pick the healthy alternative: ***apple cider vinegar.***

To produce a drink, combine:
- ✓ 2 cups of water
- ✓ 1 tablespoon of ACV

To achieve this, stir well and sip each day.

The enzymes and acetic acid in ACV normalize the acid amounts (pH amounts) of the stomach, reducing hunger pains and cravings, and producing a reduced appetite. You will find other ideas about why ACV helps regulate appetite too. One theory would be that the acetic acid in ACV reduces the glycemic index of foods, which slows the pace that sugars are released into the bloodstream, prolonging the sensation of satiety after meals and reducing cravings. Another theory would be that the pectin in ACV mixes with water/liquid and expands, resulting in a reduction in appetite. It doesn't matter how it works; it can! The very best part concerning this tonic is the fact that it's easy to create, and incredibly portable, rendering it a simple substitute for reach rather than food you'd eat and regret later.

Place a sticky note or index card on your refrigerator or cabinet where your preferred craving foods are stored, reminding you of your respective ACV appetite-suppressing option. In this manner, you start to see the reminder every time you grab foods that aren't diet-friendly.

Help Intermittent Fasting

Fasting is among the age-old, tried-and-true remedies for cleansing your body of toxins and giving yourself a "break" from a diet plan of excess. If the excess is through alcohol, fattening foods, or a standard unhealthy method of ingesting and drinking, a straightforward and easy fast which includes ACV provides a *"clean slate"* that you can begin a new method of consuming clean and living better in a matter of days.

Although some people anticipate a fast due to the natural promise that they'll feel rejuvenated, refreshed, and renewed, numerous others dread the very thought of an easy, thinking only with the feelings of starvation. If you're hesitant even to entertain the theory, *consider ACV "fasting."* It is not the same as so a great many other choices because you can still eat foods through the swift. **Paul C. Bragg** was the *"pioneer"* manufacturer and promoter of apple cider vinegar in its purest form. He used his product for maintaining health insurance and vitality and resisting illness throughout his life. He recommended an easy using his product *(Bragg's unfiltered organic ACV)* in a tonic made to flush the machine of waste, while also maintaining a strict diet of whole foods including fruits, vegetables, nuts, and seeds. By flushing the machine with fiber-rich ACV, fruits, and vegetables, the body's systems are better in a position to remove built-up waste material. In this cleanse, your body can naturally adapt to a new diet of healthy whole foods designed to keep your body free from waste by "keeping things moving."

To make Bragg's tonic, combine:

- ✓ 1 cup of water
- ✓ 1 tablespoon of ACV (or focus on ½ tablespoon and build-up to at least one 1 tablespoon)
- ✓ 1/2 tablespoon lemon juice.

Consume 3-5 instances each day for 7-10 days.

Detoxify Your Liver

Few people know very well what the liver does. The liver is an organ that secretes bile to be able to assist in effective digestion, but its responsibilities proceed far beyond that! The liver also protects and promotes one's vitality by:

- Filtering waste and waste material within the blood-producing energy by manufacturing essential proteins and storing carbohydrates along with other essential nutrients properly for metabolizing fats.

Keeping the liver free from dangerous toxins that compromise its capability to function correctly can be an essential part of maintaining general health and wellness.

You can safeguard the perfect functioning of the liver by having an eating plan and living a lifestyle that displays the liver, which has a lighter workload:
- ✓ Eat a clean diet which includes whole foods like fruits, vegetables, nuts, and seeds.
- ✓ Drink minimal alcohol.
- ✓ Drink plenty of clear fluids (preferably water).
- ✓ Avoid toxins like nicotine and drugs (prescription and otherwise).

Apple cider vinegar makes an ideal solution in liver detoxification by contributing its selection of vitamins, minerals, and enzymes to keep up a wholesome pH balance.

To produce a liver-cleansing drink, combine:
- ✓ 1 cup of water
- ✓ 1-2 teaspoons of ACV
- ✓ ½ teaspoon of raw honey.

Drink 3x a day.

Gallbladder Cleansing

The gallbladder is an organ that aids the body's systems in eliminating toxins and waste by producing the bile the liver secretes. Hand-in-hand with the liver, the gallbladder plays a significant part in maintaining a sufficient pH balance of your body, while also removing health-harming toxins. Maintaining the fitness of this organ is essential in maintaining optimal wellbeing, which explains why you should think about a flush on the gallbladder with apple cider vinegar. By performing this gallbladder cleanse twice annually, you would help your gallbladder work as intended.

To create this cleanse, combine:
- ✓ 1 cup of water
- ✓ ½ tablespoon of ACV
- ✓ 2 tablespoons of apple juice (organic, unfiltered).

Consume twice per year.

A cleanse such as this can also assist you to avoid gallstones, which are pebble-like deposits that form in the organ. Some individuals with gallstones haven't any symptoms, while some experience excruciating pain.

Gallstones are usually caused by these circumstances:
i. Once the gallbladder's bile isn't adequate enough to dissolve the liver's cholesterol production, the surplus cholesterol crystallizes and creates gallstones.
ii. If the bile contains an excessive amount of bilirubin (the consequence of the chemical break down of red blood cells).
iii. A condition referred to as cirrhosis from the liver, causing the liver to create excessive levels of bilirubin.
iv. The gallbladder's capability to vacant bile correctly is compromised, resulting in bile becoming concentrated and forming the gallstones.

Gallstones can block the passing of bile and cause extreme pain when leaving the gallbladder. Use the ACV cleanse to help avoid them significantly.

Calm Heartburn

For the incredible number of heartburn sufferers, the number of remedies (both natural and medicinal) could be overwhelming. Pills, liquids, tips about how to proceed both pre- and post-meal are enough stress to offer. Good news, forget those alternatives and instead grab ***apple cider vinegar***, which has been used to take care of heartburn for a long time. Competitors articulate there is certainly little research to aid the claim, but many people report it works like a charm. What would you lose? Nothing. Give the all-natural option a chance.

To produce a drink, combine:
- ✓ 1 cup of water
- ✓ 1 teaspoon of ACV
- ✓ 1 teaspoon of honey.

To work with, drink every thirty minutes until heartburn subsides.

The real crux in the heartburn issue may be the imbalance of acids inside the stomach, potentially due to these factors:

- The shortcoming of the body to effectively breakdown fats.

- An inadequate reaction caused by a nutrient-poor diet.
- A stomach that appears to battle foods more regularly than accepting them.

The main element of apple cider vinegar that means it is so effective in treating heartburn may be the acetic acid that results from the fermentation with the apples.

Although it seems surprising that you'll treat heartburn by introducing acid, the naturally occurring acetic acid of ACV is far weaker compared to the hydrochloric acid made by the stomach. Also, it functions as a buffer by assisting in alleviating and stopping heartburn by bringing the acidic level within the stomach to a far more normal level.

Reduce Flatulence

You can find few things as embarrassing as excessive flatulence. Embarrassing, uncomfortable, and challenging to cope with, excessive gas and flatulence is a condition that over-the-counter remedies run inside the thousands. Chemically manufactured pills and drinks that promise to lessen the incidence of gas could be effective; however, they often include countless chemicals and ingredients you can't pronounce. While myriad medical ailments could cause excessive gas, many people who experience sporadic bouts of bloating and gas can indicate processed foods as the reason. Unhealthy diets wreak havoc for the digestive system, giving excessive gas within their wake.

However, those who take in clean diets filled with fibrous roughage, such as cruciferous vegetables (broccoli, cauliflower, etc.), can have problems with excessive gas build-up and frequent flatulence. No matter what causes gas, ACV would help alleviate it. By combining a diet plan of healthy whole foods that calm gas-producing circumstances such as honey, fennel, ginger, flax, cinnamon, and pineapple with all-natural ACV tonics that treat gas, you may experience much less flatulence. The active acids and enzymes of ACV help alleviate gas production and flatulence by negating the gas-producing elements and processes involved.

To produce a tonic to take care of gas, combine:
- ✓ 1 cup of water
- ✓ 1 teaspoon of honey

- ✓ 1 teaspoon of peppermint extract
- ✓ half teaspoon of cinnamon
- ✓ 1 tablespoon of ACV

Drink daily.

Soothe stomachaches

Stomachaches could be the effect of a number of disruptions that range between psychological stresses and poor lifestyle choices to negative traits and prolonged contact with unhealthy irritants. You may experience acute stomachache occasionally, or you may be plagued with less painful but longer-lasting versions. Regardless of why you acquire stomachaches, you could effectively minimize their severity, frequency, and duration by attacking the main problem, instead of treating the symptoms. Making sure your digestive tract, from your saliva to your colon, is running effectively, you can prevent stomachaches from occurring, and treat them after they strike. By regulating the pH balance of your entire digestive tract, ACV begins fighting the sources of stomachaches. By overcoming bacteria, viruses, and possible irritants that could further exacerbate a stomachache, ACV can aid in reducing your body of possible illnesses or invaders that may cause or exacerbate uneasiness.

To produce a drink, combine:
- ✓ 1 cup of water
- ✓ 1 tablespoon of ACV.

Sip the perfect solution over an interval of thirty minutes to have rest from stomachaches.

Alleviate pregnancy morning sickness

There are always a million beautiful areas of pregnancy that just a mother can truly understand. Between watching your belly grow and feeling the flutter from the first kick, the miracle of pregnancy is awe-inspiring and joyful. One downside of pregnancy, however, may be the queasiness, nausea, or vomiting that lots of women encounter. Inaccurately known as *"morning sickness,"* this edgy feel can strike any time of the day and may range between mild to severe. As a result of varying degrees in the severe nature of morning sickness, some decide to *"ride it out."*

At the same time, some use prescription drugs for relief. While every case of morning sickness is as unique as the sufferer, *apple cider vinegar is an all-natural remedy that could assist in calming or curing morning sickness.*

To produce a morning sickness relief drink, combine:
- ✓ 2 cups of water
- ✓ ½ to 1 tablespoon of ACV
- ✓ ½ peeled part of the ginger

Sip the mixture during the period of one hour and experience relief.

ACV contains a variety of minerals and vitamins that can enhance the quality of the pregnancy by benefitting both mom and fetus, such as:
- Vitamin A, B, C, and E
- Minerals like potassium, magnesium, and iron
- Stomach-settling fibre and enzymes.

These nutrients combine to help significantly women that are pregnant:
- Regulate their body's pH balance
- Neutralize digestive enzymes, improving digestion

- Minimize bouts of diarrhea and constipation that may also contribute to morning sickness.

Relieve bouts of constipation

There is absolutely no doubt that constipation can be an unpleasant digestive condition to cope with. You might have a constant sense you need to proceed, but can't. You remain hopeful, tethered for the toilet, have problems with stomachaches and bad breath *(bad breath is a common symptom of constipation!),* plus that horrible gas and bloating! What's worse is usually that this position can pull on for over weekly. Those who find themselves on a regular pooping schedule may have the severe discomfort of constipation symptoms just a couple of hours past missing their regularly expected poop.

While several remedies can be purchased in the medicine aisles of your preferred drugstore, most of them arrive filled with chemicals, dangerous unwanted effects, or ahem, explosive results that result in a lot more pain compared to the original symptoms caused. If you need a more natural option to forcible types of constipation relief, search no further than your trusty bottle of *apple cider vinegar.*

Filled with pectin, iron, acetic acid, and fibre, ACV relieves constipation by forming a goo-like fibrous supplement within the digestive tract, helping the stool soften, form more appropriately, and move along. Like a softer, fuller stool form, many people can utilize the restroom successfully in an hour or two, naturally and without those extreme unwanted effects.

To get relief immediately, simply combine:
- ✓ 1 tablespoon of ACV
- ✓ 1 cup of water

Drink the concoction during the period of 30 minutes.

To prevent the problem from occurring again, try out this mix of treatments:
- Drink this mixture as much as 3 times daily
- Drink a lot of additional water
- Avoid caffeinated drinks
- Eat naturally fibrous whole foods like fruits, vegetables, nuts, and seeds.

Overcome Diarrhea

Diarrhea always appears to occur at most inopportune occasions. Whether you're safe in the home or at a black-tie affair, though, there is certainly never a great time to drop with this debilitating symptom. *Diarrhea is known as an indicator and not a disorder because diarrhea may be the way your body handles an unwanted aspect in the digestive tract.* If the irritant is considered a deep-fried food that isn't being appropriately digested, a virus wanting to attack the disease fighting capability, or a far more extreme case of parasites, diarrhea may be the body's natural method of promptly purging the irritant from your body and safeguarding one's health insurance and vitality. Diarrhea rids your body of the severe irritant, over the counter diarrhea medications made to quit you from heading are not the proper remedy. Whenever you ingest a formulation made to end diarrhea, it may look great for a while; nonetheless, it allows the irritant wanting to exist purged from your body to instead fester inside the digestive system all night long, wreaking havoc and perhaps spreading to other previously unaffected organs.

Medicinal remedies may also result in unintentional constipation, and this means you've simply traded one uncomfortable problem for another. *The substances in apple cider vinegar that help out with resolving diarrhea naturally are pectin, iron, and acetic acid.* These three simple elements combine to create a fibrous gel that acts as a lubricant inside the digestive tract, while also adding bulk towards the stool. What results is nothing in short supply of a miracle cure! In only 30 mins, ACV moves waste quickly through the body system, but in a way that is a lot more comfortable than previously experienced.

To produce a drink to solve diarrhea, combine:
- ✓ 1 cup tepid to warm water
- ✓ 1-2 tablespoons of ACV.

Drink the mixture over an interval of quarter-hour. It is safe to take this concoction repeatedly every hour before diarrhea subsides.

Avoid Bacterial Cystitis (UTI)

*Bacterial cystitis is a medical term that's used interchangeably using the better-known term "urinary system infection" or **UTI**.* Cystitis is thought of as an inflammation in the bladder, mostly due to bacteria. The choice for the bacterial cause is interstitial cystitis. The bacterial version of cystitis additionally occurs in women; nonetheless, it may also be experienced by men and children; women are particularly vulnerable to the problem for their shorter urethras, which are more easily subjected to harmful bacteria.

The problem starts just like a tingling sensation and will then become severe, with symptoms that cause the sufferer to feel the frequent urge to urinate, with or without urine being expelled, and include pain and burning sensations experienced during urination. Since bacterial cystitis is a bacterial infection with the bladder, antibiotics will be the standard treatment. However, natural methods may be used to prevent and alleviate the problem.

Filled with valuable minerals and vitamins that help out with flushing your body of poisons like the parasites that contribute to this uncomfortable condition, *apple cider vinegar produces an ideal preventive option in stopping bacterial cystitis before it starts.* You will find two methods to do that:

To produce a drink, combine:
- ✓ 1 cup of water
- ✓ 1 tablespoon of ACV.

Drink daily.

Many women report experiencing fewer incidences of bacterial cystitis before they start an ACV routine, plus they experienced a lower life expectancy severity in symptoms if they consumed the concoction following the onset of the problem.

You can even try out this bathing method:

Combine inside a bathtub:
- ✓ 1 cup ACV
- ✓ A tub filled with warm water

Soak for thirty minutes.

This bath alleviates symptoms by killing bacteria within the urethra.

Limit Interstitial Cystitis

While bacterial cystitis can be a commonly experienced infection that triggers inflammation on the bladder, interstitial cystitis is often a persistent condition seen as inflammation from the submucosal and muscular layers in the bladder. Sometimes known as bladder pain syndrome, or BPS, interstitial cystitis is seen as a severe symptom such as blood inside the urine, intense pelvic pain, as well as the sudden urge to urinate (with or without urine being excreted) around sixty times each day. Probably the most daunting facet of this condition is the fact that it does not have any known cause or no known cure. Doctors remain stumped concerning if the condition is hereditary, a congenital disability, because of vascular disease, or frustrated by allergies.

Without a known cure for the problem, many sufferers are forced to endure the pain with no treatment, or within the most unfortunate cases, have the bladder removed. Some interstitial cystitis sufferers choose preventive measures they can take from home. They cautiously know what physical, diet, or environmental factors contribute to their flare-ups of the problem. *Since there is no cure, interstitial cystitis shows to improve using the restricting of particular foods and drinks like sodas, caffeinated beverages, and citric fruits and drinks.* Furthermore, to restricting aggravating dietary elements, *apple cider vinegar can help to calm the problem by:*

- Providing nutrients that assist the bladder in processing urine
- Minimizing the toxicity in the urine
- Detoxifying the blood and body fluids that play a role inside the bladder's functioning.

You can introduce ACV into the body through this simple, versatile tonic:

To produce a drink, combine:

- ✓ 1 cup of water
- ✓ 1 tablespoon of ACV

Consume the beverage during the period of thirty minutes, and continue steadily to drink the same combination every hour until symptoms subside.

Minimize Iron Insufficiency

Iron insufficiency is thought of as an inadequate way to obtain red blood cells, which leads to tissues being deprived of essential oxygen. *Common symptoms are extreme fatigue and weakness.* And a short way to obtain red blood cells, the body's failure to create enough red blood cells or excessive bleeding (even heavy menstrual flows can qualify as excessive bleeding) is usually to blame. Although some symptoms of iron insufficiency (also called *iron-deficiency anaemia*) are mild enough, they can move unnoticed for an extended time frame; many anaemia symptoms are powerful enough to improve one's day-to-day life dramatically.

Once the body's capability to absorb and utilize enough iron is compromised, lots of the body's systems are affected, and the effect is as wide as several symptoms, such as:

- Fatigue
- Mood swings
- A compromised disease fighting capability.

By firmly taking an over-the-counter iron supplement, you can moderate iron insufficiency. However, by taking ACV day-by-day, you can help in iron absorption and decrease the dependence on supplements frequently.

To create an iron-boosting drink, combine:
- ✓ 2 cups of water
- ✓ 2 tablespoons of ACV
- ✓ ½ cup of spinach
- ✓ ½ green apple, cored.

Combine all ingredients inside a blender and blend until thoroughly combined.
Drink daily.

Increase Calcium Absorption

Some people assume they know the need for calcium; few know the profound effects this essential mineral is wearing several systems in the torso. One of the most well-known roles of calcium is building and maintaining healthy bones and teeth, and indeed, 99% of the body's calcium is stored in the bones and teeth. What few people know, though, can be that essential mineral can be valuable for:

- Cognition
- Proper nervous system functioning
- Maintaining muscle tissue
- Preventing blood circulation
- Pressure issues.

Certainly, with regards to maintaining one's general health, calcium is among the most important nutrients. Challenging supplements and calcium-fortified products obtainable, you might be beneath the impression that you're getting enough of the magical mineral in what you eat, but you might be mistaken. *While supplements can help, a diet plan, including calcium-rich foods-including* **apple cider vinegar***, is the ultimate way to consume calcium.*

Surprisingly enough, a more natural way to make sure you're absorbing probably the most calcium from your foods is undoubtedly to start an apple cider vinegar program that may contribute two essentials with a need to maximize calcium absorption from the foods you take in each day: *acetic acid and magnesium.* The acetic acid that's within ACV promotes the body's absorption of calcium by assisting in the wearing down of calcium-rich foods and aiding digestion. Calcium-rich foods like deep-green veggies contain compounds called oxalates that truly block calcium absorption.

The acetic acid in ACV neutralizes these oxalates and makes the ingested calcium easier absorbed. As well as acetic acid, ACV also includes magnesium, which supports calcium absorption.

To produce a drink that supports calcium absorption, combine:

- 1 cup of calcium-fortified orange juice
- 1 tablespoon of ACV.

Drink daily.

Avoid Vitamin C Deficiencies

When a person is in good general health, each of your respective body's systems can function at its full capability. Many people have problems with ailments when their disease fighting capability is usually compromised. Whether it's a common cold, vitamin or mineral deficiency, or even more severe health issue, you become vulnerable to several other health threats if your disease fighting capability isn't working correctly. Even prescriptions and over-the-counter medications can compromise the immune system's capability to fight disruptions inside the body's natural balances of minerals, fluids, and bacteria; this example is often seen when antibiotics get rid of the illness intended but promote the growth of parasites that results in yeast-based infections. Certainly, once the body's systems are operating better, and synergistically, your disease fighting capability functions significantly! You understand, given that apple cider vinegar provides essential vitamins, minerals, and enzymes. Also, it offers antiviral and antibacterial houses that combine to aid the disease fighting capability in fighting illnesses while also ensuring your body functions at optimal levels. This optimal functioning includes absorbing essential dietary nutrients and utilizing them better.

Apple cider vinegar contains vitamin C and can help you absorb it better too. By drinking ACV, you may kick-start an advantageous cycle that improves the body's immunity, enables your body to raised absorb the vitamin, improving immunity, etc.

To produce a daily vitamin c-boosting drink, combine:
- ✓ 1 cup of organic apple juice
- ✓ 1 frozen banana
- ✓ 1 cup of frozen strawberries
- ✓ 1 teaspoon of cinnamon
- ✓ 1 tablespoon of ACV.

Combine all ingredients within a blender and blend until desired consistency is achieved. Enjoy once daily.

Avoid Vitamin-B Deficiencies

Vitamin-B is in charge of ensuring the correct functioning of any surprising number of systems. B-vitamins play a significant role in the body's general health, including:

- Maintaining a positive mindset (vitamin B deficiencies are connected with depression)
- Promoting proper protein synthesis
- Nourishing nerve cells

- Offering the fundamental elements for DNA synthesis.

Surprisingly enough, many people are unaware of how exactly to include even more B vitamin-rich foods within their diet to avoid experiencing a B-vitamin deficiency. *Foods such as nut products, seeds, avocados, spinach, peas, asparagus, mushrooms, and spirulina certainly are an excellent addition to any B-vitamin-deficient diet.* The next ACV tonic may also assist you in making sure your vitamin B levels remain safe and stable. *Spirulina can be a supplemental alga powder that's readily available generally in most health food stores and several local food markets.*

To produce a drink, combine:
- ✓ 1 tablespoon of ACV
- ✓ 1 cup of water
- ✓ 1 teaspoon of spirulina
- ✓ 1 pear, cored.

Combine all ingredients inside a blender (with ice if desired) and blend until desired consistency is achieved. Drink daily.

Each B vitamin plays another role in assisting the body:

- **B (thiamine)**: Involved in the formation of vigor from carbohydrates and RNA and DNA production. *Deficiency results in neurological complications, pain, and sensory issues.*
- **B (riboflavin)**: Aids in energy production for electrolyte transport, and it is mixed up in the transformation of fatty-acid molecules into energy. *Deficiency contributes to ariboflavinosis, where cracked lips, sensitivity to sunlight, and a sore throat result in more severe health issues.*
- **B (niacin)**: Involved inside the energy-transfer reactions within the metabolism of glucose, fat, and alcohol. *Deficiency can lead to aggression, insomnia, weakness, and dermatitis.*
- **B (pantothenic acid)**: Involved inside the oxidation of essential fatty acids and carbs, as well as the formation of amino acids, essential fatty acids, ketones, cholesterol, and steroid hormones. *The most frequent sign of deficiency is acne.*
- **B (pyridoxine)**: Involved within the metabolism of proteins and lipids, and the formation of

neurotransmitters and haemoglobin. *Deficiency leads to microcytic anaemia, depression, dermatitis, hypertension, and fluid retention.*

- **B (biotin)**: Involved inside the metabolism of lipids, proteins, and carbohydrates and metabolizing energy, proteins, and cholesterol. *Deficiency brings about impaired growth and neurological disorders in infants.*

- **B (folic acid):** Ensures normal cell division, especially during pregnancy, and plays a significant role in the production of red blood cells. *Deficiency results in high degrees of homocysteine and may result in delivery problems.*

- **B (various cobalamins)**: Involved in the cell metabolism of carbohydrates, proteins, and lipids, and the production of red blood cells in bone marrow, nerve sheaths, and proteins. *Deficiency results in memory loss and cognitive defects.*

Irritable Bowel Syndrome (IBS)

Irritable bowel syndrome (IBS) is seen as uncomfortable digestion because of pain familiar with the intestinal muscle spasms necessary for moving food with the colon. As well as the pain experienced from the procedure of digestion, those that endure IBS also experience diarrhea, constipation, or both, frequently. *IBS does not have any known cause, plus the treatments for the problem range from natural to pharmaceutical and number in the hundreds.*

As with many of the pharmaceutical answers to medical conditions, the medicines created to treat IBS have certain undesirable side effects that have prompted IBS sufferers to seek more natural alternatives. With specific acids that neutralize digestive enzymes and stomach acid, pectin for a fiber that softens and bulks stools for easier passage through the colon, and antiviral and antibacterial properties that help to maintain an optimal balance of bacteria in the gut, *apple cider vinegar is growing in popularity as a natural IBS pain reliever.* Packed with beneficial vitamins, minerals, enzymes, and natural phytochemicals that act to protect your immunity on a cellular level, ACV is not only an inexpensive and easily attainable remedy; it's simple to integrate into any lifestyle.

To produce a preventive tonic, combine:
- ✓ 1 tablespoon of ACV
- ✓ 2 cups of water

Sip the concoction ahead of meals to help significantly prevent IBS.

To produce a tonic to help current symptoms, combine greatly:
- ✓ 2-4 teaspoons of ACV
- ✓ 1 cup of water

Sip during the period of 30 minutes.

Enhance a Vegetarian Diet Plan

The most frequent risk connected with a vegetarian diet plan is the chance for passing up on certain essential nutrients that needed to optimize the body's functioning. There are always a handful of specific vegetarian groups that are categorized with what is usually avoided within their diets:

- *A "vegetarian" (who eats no meat, but includes milk products, eggs, and animal products).*
- *A "vegan" (who avoids all products produced from animals).*

Vegetarian and vegan diets that exclude meat and animal products are certainly in a position to supply the essential micronutrients our anatomies need.

By planning vegetarian or vegan meals offering all the necessary minerals and vitamins, you could meet all dietary needs.

Adding apple cider vinegar to a vegetarian or vegan diet supplies the following benefits:

- It supports the absorption of macronutrients (carbohydrates, proteins, and fats) and micronutrients consumed within the daily food diet. With this optimized absorption, amino acid absorption and processing can be optimized, ensuring proper cell functioning and growth.

- The fibre naturally occurring in ACV supports digestion, reducing difficult digestion issues commonly from the plant-based foods contained in the vegetarian diet plan. Naturally occurring phytonutrients, as well as enzymes containing antiviral and antibacterial properties, are also contained in ACV, boosting the immune system of a vegetarian diet plan (which may be without immunity-boosting vitamins typically within milk products and healthy meat).

To produce a calcium-boosting drink, combine within a blender:

- ✓ ½ tablespoon of ACV
- ✓ 1 cup of coconut or almond milk
- ✓ Your preferred fruits and spices

Drink daily.

Chapter 5
ACV For Complete Wellness

When you have nature's medicine cabinet by optimizing your daily diet and focusing your regular consumption of foods on natural, whole varieties, you will maximize your overall health and wellness by naturally supplying ample amounts of essential vitamins, minerals, and protective elements. *This is a well-known fact.* When you suffer from medical conditions and health-depleting illnesses, it can be easy to fall victim to the marketing ploys that drug manufacturers spend billions of dollars to design to ensure that you choose their products for calming symptoms or curing ailments.

But, if you prefer to seek out natural treatments over the pharmaceutically produced pills and potions that promise to cure illnesses and relieve symptoms, you are one of the millions of consumers who have decided to turn to nature for better health! Not only can apple cider vinegar provide you with relief from common life-altering symptoms; it can improve your overall health and return you to the quality of life you dream of. Many health conditions result from damage to the body's cells, deficiencies of nutrients needed for optimal system functioning, or extensive multisystem dysfunction that results in a domino-effect-like series of illnesses. Whether you have diabetes and poor circulation, chronic inflammation and muscle stiffness, or even depression and anxiety, you can easily find yourself in a seemingly unpredictable manner of ill health.

The glad tidings are that whenever you get the systems back on the right track, focus your way of life and diet on healthy activities and whole foods, and implement a straightforward ACV regimen within your day to day routine; you can take control of your health and get back to living naturally! Vitamin deficiencies can wreak havoc on your body by affecting the functioning of one system that affects another and another and so on, leading to a breakdown in multiple areas of the body. If you consider the body as parts of a whole, you can see why it's necessary to not simply treat just one symptom or one illness but rather treat the body as an integrative series of systems functioning to assist and support each other. By ensuring your body is receiving quality nutrients that provide all of the body's systems with ample supplies of what they need, you can remedy not one but many health issues at the same time.

Detoxify The Natural Way

Apple cider vinegar is used as a highly useful detoxification tool, as well as for a good reason!

The primary goals of your detox are to:

- Cleanse the machine of toxins, such as air and environmental pollutants, processed ingredients from foods, and chemicals from everyday products.
- Assist the body's organ systems in ridding your body of built-up waste.
- Replenish the body's stores of valuable minerals and vitamins needed for optimal functioning.

An apple cider vinegar detox offers many of these benefits, and much more, making it an ideal addition to a detoxification plan. It's simple, secure, and effective, and certain to leave you feeling rejuvenated, refreshed, and healthfully replenished! An all-natural, organic option that provides a number of vitamins, minerals, and essential nutrients, ACV could be the perfect supplement that gives cleansing properties and restorative minerals and vitamins, all you need to make sure you're providing the body with what it needs during a detoxification program.

To Produce A Supplemental Detox Drink, Combine:
- ✓ 1 tablespoon of ACV
- ✓ 2 cups of water

Drink the ACV mixture each day, afternoon, and evening. In case your detox includes meals, drink the mixture thirty minutes ahead of meals.

An average detoxification plan lasts for you to a week and sometimes includes whole foods. Usually, you begin by consuming only liquids; you then might slowly introduce whole foods. Some people choose to make use of a liquid-only cleanse to be able to permit the body to rid itself of waste and begin "fresh" till the detox is completed, there exists a significant benefit in including certain whole foods: Adding fibre will help the body's digestive tract in purging waste.

A detox plan which includes ACV provides so many advantages:

- Beneficial enzymes and acetic acid that help neutralize stomach acids.
- Added fibre, which forms a gel inside the gut and helps to remove toxins and waste, helps the liver (along with other organs that perform essential roles in detoxifying the body) effectively remove toxins while replenishing stores of vitamins and minerals needed to operate more effectively.
- Powerful antioxidants that boost the immune system and safeguard one's health throughout the detoxification process.

Many people who consume ACV have reported a boost in energy levels, which becomes essential during any fast.

Improve A Diabetic Lifestyle

People with diabetes focus a lot of their attention to eating foods offering quality nutrition and help out with maintaining stable blood sugar. Even though many people with diabetes discover this dietary focus just a little overwhelming when getting started, the procedure of selecting specific foods that are diabetes-friendly becomes second nature quickly enough. Whether or not you have been diagnosed as prediabetic or is a verified type 1 or type 2 diabetic, many patients struggling with diabetic symptoms can find relief by simply adding apple cider vinegar to their daily diet regimen. Packed with enzymes and acetic acid that aid in maintaining the body's blood glucose levels at optimal numbers for longer durations, apple cider vinegar has shown to improve the diabetic lifestyle in the following ways:

- Reducing the frequency of blood sugar levels spikes and dips.
- Providing a sense of fullness lasting long following the completion of meals, diabetics also report consuming a far more standard diet of smaller, more frequent meals, causing an even more stable blood glucose level.
- Helping diabetics experience less frequent bouts of diarrhea and constipation that may be derived from the diabetic diet or medications prescribed to manage the condition.

The fast-acting acetic acid and pectin in ACV help the body's digestive system maintain normal functioning by adding bulk to stools and lubricating the digestive system to move waste more effectively.

As ACV makes a difference in potassium and magnesium levels, it's vital that you speak to your doctor about whether ACV may be right for you.

If so, try out this tonic:

- ✓ 2 teaspoons of ACV
- ✓ ½ cup organic, unfiltered apple juice
- ✓ 1 cup of water

Consume the mixture upon rising each day, ahead of breakfast, and ahead of bedtime.

Help Safeguard against Cancer

Cancer is among the most dreadful diseases of contemporary times. Cancers of most types affect people of every gender, age, and ethnicity. While there are known factors that contribute to the introduction of cancer cells- such as genetics, sun exposure, smoking, as well as other environmental and lifestyle factors, sometimes, there's no warning. Cancer treatments include many severe adverse effects that vary from hair loss to extreme nausea and fatigue. Due to the increasing awareness of cancer and its treatments, many people are looking for natural preventive measures that can be taken in an attempt to safeguard their health from cancerous developments. *One such natural method is vitamin C. Though it may seem like a simple vitamin couldn't possibly affect a disease as serious as cancer, it can.*

Vitamin C can influence cancer in the following ways:
- Acts as a robust antioxidant that may finish cancerous changes within cells by reversing the damage done by free radicals that cause the cancerous changes.
- Vitamin C infusions show to drastically enhance the general health of some cancer patients, improving the potency of cancer treatments and helping some patients reach the idea of remission.
- It improves the potency of the disease fighting capability. It helps with the body's capability to absorb the essential vitamins and minerals required to function correctly.

For a glass or two that will help boost vitamin C levels, combine these ingredients inside a blender until desired consistency is reached:

- ✓ 1 cup of freshly squeezed orange juice
- ✓ 1/2 cup of freshly squeezed grapefruit juice
- ✓ 1 tablespoon of ACV
- ✓ 1 frozen banana

Drink daily.

End The Hiccups

You can find seemingly, an incredible number of theories about how exactly or why we get hiccups and as many theories of how exactly to cure them. Medically, one of the most accepted theories in regards to what happens throughout an episode of the hiccups is usually a repetitive spasm on the diaphragm. The diaphragm is a dome-shaped muscle separating the chest through the abdomen, along with the spasm occurring within the diaphragm causes an immediate reactive closure from the vocal cords, creating the "hiccup" sound.

While the hiccups are a harmless condition, they can be very annoying, and in some cases, very uncomfortable.

While, for most people, the hiccups generally lasts for only a few minutes, there have been reported cases of hiccups lasting for days, weeks, and even months! Whether the cause is nerves, eating or drinking too fast, or the body's natural attempt to deliver more oxygen to the brain, the hiccups are one more condition that apple cider vinegar can help! Due to its strong taste, pungent aroma, and powerful effects within the digestive system, apple cider vinegar causes immediate physical reactions that many people credit in its effectiveness as a cure for hiccups. While the medical support for ACV as a cure for hiccups may not be available just yet, decades and generations of avid ACV users are happy to attest to the effectiveness as a hiccup cure. *What do you have to lose? Nothing.*

To produce a drink, combine:
- ✓ 1 tablespoon of ACV
- ✓ 1 cup of water

Consume between hiccups.

Relieve Muscle Stiffness

Lactic acid may be the normal byproduct made by muscles following the processing of essential proteins. The build-up of lactic acid inside the muscles is the cause of tightness and pain in areas like the neck, back, butt, legs, and arms. While stretching may be the best approach to cure muscle stiffness, because it allows the muscles to release the lactic acid into the blood to become carried away as waste, many muscle stiffness sufferers opt for over-the-counter treatments. Unfortunately, most relieve the pain only temporarily, and in some cases, even aggravate the condition! Luckily, the lactic acid build-up in the muscles can be naturally treated by stretching of the thickened areas and using various apple cider vinegar applications.

ACV contains acetic acid and vitamins and minerals that aid in the processing of elements such as lactic acid.

To produce a drink, combine:
- ✓ 1 cup of water
- ✓ 2 teaspoons of ACV

Drink daily.

To produce a soothing bath, combine:
- ✓ A tub filled with normal water
- ✓ 2 cups of ACV

Soaking for thirty minutes allows the nutrients, acids, and enzymes in ACV to pull toxins from your body, enabling your body to better clear the muscles and blood of lactic acid build-up.

Get Rid of a Stuffy Nose

If the cause is allergies, a typical cold, or perhaps a vicious virus, a stuffy nose can be an awful symptom to see. Cleverly created marketing strategies are made to bombard stuffy-nose-sufferers using the temptation of relief within a bottle. Desperate consumers choose these quick fixes in the height of cold and flu or allergy seasons, unknowingly getting more than they bargained for. Pills, drinks, and sprays that act to unstuff a stuffy nose are made using combinations of steroids, stimulants, and chemicals that aid in drying up the nose.

While these over-the-counter treatments can be effective, the majority of them contain potent ingredients that produce harmful side effects that can wreak havoc on your body and mind. From jitters and endless energy to symptoms that return right away, over-the-counter remedies can be more hazardous than helpful. This is just one of the reasons consumers are turning to natural remedies instead of pharmaceutically created options. *Apple cider vinegar is one of the tried-and-true natural alternatives that have been used to clear up stuffy noses for centuries.* All it takes is a sniff of apple cider vinegar to experience the effectiveness of the tonic's ability to clear the sinuses! The enzymes and antiviral properties contained in ACV can be useful in relieving a stuffy nose in three ways:

To produce a drink, combine:
- ✓ 1 tablespoon of ACV
- ✓ 1 cup of warm water

Drink to relieve symptoms.

To produce a steam treatment, boil:
- ✓ 4 cups of water

✓ 1 cup of ACV

Simply drape a towel over your mind while you lean on the pot to trap the steam. Inhale the vapors.

To utilize an ACV tonic like a neti pot fluid, combine:
1 cup of water
2 teaspoons of ACV
To utilize, drain down the sinuses and from the throat.

Ease a Sore Throat

A sore throat will come on unexpectedly and will be an isolated experience or an indicator of the much more severe condition. Pharyngitis, meaning "inflammation in the throat," maybe the medical term for any sore throat. Although it has a number of causes that vary from infection to irritation, a sore throat must be treated as soon as the scratchiness, irritation, and pain arise. *Whether the crux of the issue is viral or bacterial, apple cider vinegar is a natural remedy that provides nutritional benefits that calm from the inside out.*

Containing several naturally occurring vitamins, minerals, enzymes, and antioxidants along with antiviral and antibiotic properties that work together in soothing a sore throat, ACV in its natural, unfiltered, organic state can perform the job of many medications all on its own!

To produce a drink, combine:

- ✓ 1 cup of warmed water
- ✓ 1 tablespoon of ACV
- ✓ 1 teaspoon of honey (if developing a tonic to drink)

Gargle the mixture by cup gulps, or drink the tonic warmed using the added teaspoon of honey to kill germs in the mouth and throat when you swallow the mixture.

The vitamin C within ACV also provides immunity-boosting effects by fending off illness while also strengthening the disease fighting capability.

Soothe Sinusitis

Sinusitis, also called a sinus infection, is a condition of the effect of a microorganism (using a bacteria, virus, or fungus) that grows in the air pockets with the sinus and causes a blockage. Although some experience sinusitis occasionally, many sufferers find out they have got chronic sinus problems. Due to *Chlamydia*, the sinuses swell and commence producing an abnormal amount of mucus.

As *Chlamydia* persists, the inflammation and mucus cause the original sinusitis symptoms of headaches, facial tenderness, sinus pressure and pain, fever, dark and cloudy nasal discharge, stuffiness, sore throat, cough, as well as toothaches. Even though many cases of sinusitis require antibiotics, some sinusitis sufferers will get relief a long time before *Chlamydia* continues to grow to the idea of requiring prescribed drugs. Over-the-counter relievers work in soothing sore throats, relieving pain and fevers, and drying up mucus; however, they may also deliver unwanted effects. For sinusitis sufferers choosing to use natural treatments before embracing considerably more extreme measures, apple cider vinegar may be the perfect option. *Containing antibacterial and antiviral properties, apple cider vinegar is filled with essential antioxidants, vitamins, and minerals that combine to combat infections and soothe symptoms.* Reinforcing the body's disease-fighting capability with plenty of natural vitamin C, ACV provides support to some sinusitis sufferer by alleviating the symptoms, pinpointing the reason for the problem, and boosting the disease fighting capability.

To produce a soothing drink to combat the foundation of sinusitis (bacterial, viral, or others), combine:
- ✓ 1 tablespoon of ACV •
- ✓ 1 cup of warm water

Drink 3 times daily.

To produce a steam treatment, combine within a pot:
- ✓ 1 cup of ACV
- ✓ 4 cups of water

Inhale the vapors as the steam is produced.

Combat High Cholesterol

Many people are unaware that cholesterol is genuinely a positive thing that your body needs to be able to function correctly. Cholesterol helps your body produce and process vitamin D, digestive bile, and several hormones. Cholesterol is ever-present within the blood in case of a problem when there exists an excessive amount of this "positive thing." Adding to the introduction of severe conditions like cardiovascular disease and stroke, uncontrolled cholesterol amounts can lead to serious health issues and complications. Made up of several factors like the degrees of LDL (the "bad" cholesterol), HDL (the "high" cholesterol), and triglycerides inside the blood, your cholesterol levels could be checked with a straightforward blood test that determines when you have healthy or unhealthy levels. Several factors, including age, genealogy, diet, and lifestyle habits (smoking, alcohol consumption, etc.) can all play a role in affecting cholesterol amounts. By taking a dynamic role in minimizing the contributing factors to raised cholesterol amounts, you can lessen your threat of developing the dangerous condition. Packed with magnesium, potassium, vitamins A, B, and C, and several enzymes that help out with maintaining general health, *apple cider vinegar also has a crucial element called pectin that helps your body rid itself of excess cholesterol.* **Pectin** *binds to excess cholesterol within the digestive tract and transports it from the body as waste. By detaching excess cholesterol, your body experiences a wholesome degree of cholesterols and may better maintain those levels.*

To produce a cholesterol combating tonic, combine:
- ✓ 1 teaspoon of ACV
- ✓ 1 cup of water

Drink twice daily.

Much like most medical issues, there are a variety of prescription drugs available for treating high blood circulation pressure. Much like most medications, though, they often come with undesired side effects that may severely impact your day-to-day life. Due to the serious unwanted effects of drugs, many people are choosing to attempt to treat their high blood circulation pressure more naturally. Speak to your doctor in what strategy is right for you.

Reduce Bad Breath

Everyone gets bad breath occasionally. It could be because of several factors, such as diet, hygiene, and lifestyle habits such as smoking. Although some cases of bad breath will be the consequence of severe illnesses and health issues, the common cause of bad breath is because of germs in the mouth and throat. Brushing your teeth regularly and utilizing a mouthwash might seem such as a perfect solution for bad breath, however when it involves killing germs, products available in the market are occasionally ineffective, and most contain harsh chemicals that can be questionable for consumption.

Check the label on yours; you might see warnings like "usually do not swallow" or "not safe for consumption"! That warning probably enables you to reconsider the over-the-counter bad breath remedies and decide on an even more natural solution. *Apple cider vinegar provides antiviral, antibacterial, and antiseptic properties, and therefore works well in killing viruses, bacteria, and germs. Apple cider vinegar's capability to kill the bacteria and germs inside the mouth, on one's teeth, and in the gums helps it be an ideal solution.*

A significant note: Due to the effectiveness of the acids in ACV, it is unsafe to take undiluted (to be able to protect one's teeth from being stripped of the protective enamel). Diluted, though, this natural do-it-yourself solution could be used like a mouth rinse and a gargle to kill from the bad-breath-causing germs and bacteria effectively.

To produce a mouth rinse, combine:
- ✓ 2 teaspoons of ACV
- ✓ ½ cup of water

Swish in the mouth for 15-20 seconds before spitting.

To produce a gargle, combine:
- ✓ 2 teaspoons of ACV
- ✓ ½ cup of water

Gargle the mixture for 20-30 seconds at the same time, typically repeat as necessary.

Fight Exhaustion

You have, without a doubt, experienced "normal" exhaustion, for example, when you've undergone strenuous activity for long durations, had extensive contact with heat, or endured excessive hours without sleep. "Abnormal" exhaustion is known to get feelings of fatigue if the sufferer has engaged in no such strenuous activity or is not subjected to environmental factors that could contribute to exhaustive feelings. If the exhaustive experience is acute or chronic, many sufferers consider everyday remedies such as caffeinated drinks like tea or coffee, or even more extreme over-the-counter stimulants.

Coffees and teas are occasionally effective in suddenly stimulating the senses and so are deemed safe as well as sometimes good for one's general health; however, they provide only a temporary solution accompanied by an accident that leads to returning to the initial state of exhaustion. *For all those experiencing exhaustion frequently, apple cider vinegar offers benefits that target several areas serving to treat the issue safely and naturally using its abundant naturally occurring nutrients and enzymes that improve energy, mental stability, cognitive functioning, nerve functioning, and metabolic functioning!* How?

Packed with natural vitamins like B and C, apple cider vinegar can enhance the body's strength naturally by stimulating the mind, muscles, and tissues without causing jittery or restless symptoms. ACV offers have been shown to enhance the systems that directly affect energy (nervous system for cognition and mental clarity, disease fighting capability for general health maintenance, and metabolism for energy and stamina, to mention several).

The antioxidants within ACV help out with the repair on the body's cells, aiding in feelings of refreshment and rejuvenation. ACV's selection of beneficial minerals and vitamins replenish depleted stores of the essentials and boost disease fighting capability functioning.

To create an energy-boosting tonic, combine:
- ✓ 1 tablespoon of ACV
- ✓ 2 cups of water
- ✓ ½ cup freshly squeezed orange juice

Consume the mixture 3 x daily.

Overcome Laryngitis

By eating apple cider vinegar, you can deliver antiviral, antibacterial, antifungal, and antiseptic properties contained within ACV towards the larynx. The next concoctions can offer relief for the irritated area, as the germ-fighting houses kill the resources of irritation, leaving the larynx free from irritants and better fitted to recovery.

To produce a drink, combine:

- ✓ 1 cup tepid to warm water
- ✓ 1 tablespoon of ACV
- ✓ 1 teaspoon of organic honey

Drink every 30-60 minutes until symptoms subside.

To produce a gargle, combine:

- ✓ ½ cup of hot water
- ✓ 2-4 tablespoons of ACV

Gargle the mixture for 20-30 seconds at the same time, typically repeat as necessary.

The gargle can prevent further irritation due to looming germs, toxins, and dust on one's teeth, tongue, gums, and throat; gargling with this solution also minimizes further irritation from postnasal drips that may seep down the back from the throat. Whether you have problems with allergies, have inhaled environmental toxins, or are coping with a cold or flu, laryngitis will probably be your body's reaction to irritants within the larynx. Natural treatments for resolving laryngitis and calming the symptoms that result have become increasingly more appealing, as pharmaceutical companies continue steadily to use chemicals and harsh additions within their treatments. Through the use of apple cider vinegar as a cure, one will discover the relief of laryngitis naturally, and without the undesirable unwanted effects that may sometimes accompany over-the-counter medications.

Relieve Leg Pain

Cramps inside the muscles through the entire body could be due to issues such as:

- Nutrient deficiencies
- Dehydration
- Excessive deterioration caused by exercise or bouts of Physical endurance
- Poor circulation.

If the leg cramps you have derive from these possible causes or appear to have been due to another factor, your neighbourhood pharmacy probably has a vast selection of anti-inflammatory pills, tonics, and skin medications that promise to supply relief. Even though many of the solutions could be useful, they could provide only a temporary respite and often feature a host of possible undesirable unwanted effects.

When you are experiencing leg cramps, try these ACV options.

To produce a quick-acting tonic, combine:
- ✓ 1 tablespoon of ACV
- ✓ 2 cups of water

Drink 1-3 times daily until symptoms subside.

To produce a soothing bath solvent, combine:
- ✓ A tub filled with tepid to warm water
- ✓ 1 cup of ACV.

Soak within the mixture for 30 minutes to alleviate lactic acid build-up, stimulate circulation, and remove toxins.

The organic, unfiltered variety can replenish the body's stores of valuable minerals and vitamins that are usually depleted when cramping and muscle soreness occur.

To produce a topical solution, dampen a wet towel with ACV.

Apply the towel right to the cramping section of the leg to alleviate lactic acid buildup, stimulate circulation, and remove toxins.

Apple cider vinegar contains several reparative minerals and vitamins which have been proven to provide treatment in muscles and joints. Thought to improve circulation in the blood, ACV is used to ease muscle cramping and soreness by stimulating blood circulation through the entire body and delivering higher volumes of oxygenated blood towards the areas in need.

Reduces the Chance of Cataracts

Quality eyesight is key to nearly every facet of everyday living. Taking the steps essential to safeguard your eye health now will make sure you can continue enjoying pursuits like reading, sports, and driving for a long time to come. Probably one of the most commonly experienced eye-related issues is cataracts, which condition could be helped or hindered by the approach to life choices you make each day. The light that enters your eye passes via a lens directly behind your iris, so when the oxidative stress of free radicals damages the cells with this lens, the natural proteins with the lens clump together and make the lens cloudy, hardened, and discoloured.

This is what we refer to as a cataract. Because free radicals are at fault in causing the cell damage leading to cataracts, the simplest way to avoid and reverse harm to the eye's lens is usually to include as many antioxidant-rich foods in the dietary plan as you possibly can. A diet plan of fruits and vegetables abundant with antioxidants-along with ACV- can support your eyes to remain healthy. *Apple cider vinegar:* Supplies the antioxidants which combat oxidative stress that directly affects eye health
Contains beta carotene, probably one of the essential nutrients for eye health, and supports the regeneration of cells inside the eyes while safeguarding those same cells from further damage.

To create an eye-health-friendly drink, combine:
- ✓ 1 cup of fresh carrot juice

- ✓ Juice of ½ ginger
- ✓ 1 tablespoon of ACV

Drink daily.

Alleviate Foot Fungus

Not merely is foot fungus an uncomfortable condition; it could be very uncomfortable and challenging to cure. While you will find loads of over-the-counter antifungal creams and powerful prescriptions made to cope with the unsightly condition, most are costly, ineffective, or provide as many uncomfortable unwanted effects because they do results. As more natural alternatives to chemical-laden options become increasingly appealing, apple cider vinegar has turned into a popular recommendation for treating foot fungus. In its raw, unfiltered form, apple cider vinegar has been shown to alleviate skin conditions like foot fungus in two ways: internally and on-site, rendering it effective as a cure and also being a preventive measure.

To produce a drink that improves the body's disease fighting capability, combine:

- ✓ 1 tablespoon of ACV
- ✓ 1 cup of water

Drink the concoction daily.

This drink has antiseptic properties that induce a wholesome environment where fungi have less chance for growth.

To produce a localized treatment, soak a little towel with ACV.

Apply on the affected area for thirty minutes at the same time.

The antifungal properties within ACV combat the growth on the fungus and stop the problem from spreading.

Reduce Asthma Symptoms

The vitamin C in ACV could be harnessed to take care of the symptoms of asthma effectively and without side effects by giving the beneficial vitamins necessary for improved immunity and eased respiratory functioning without chemicals or additives. How? ACV improves the immune system using vitamin C and antioxidants. With a far more effective disease fighting capability, people living with asthma will be able to fight better certain triggers, such as environmental irritants, common colds, and respiratory infections. The inhaled and applied treatments using ACV also be effective in reducing the incidence and severity of asthma symptoms.

To produce a drink, combine:
- ✓ 1 tablespoon of ACV
- ✓ ½ cup of freshly juiced ginger
- ✓ 1 cup of water

Drink daily.

To produce a steam treatment, boil inside a pot:
- ✓ 4 cups of water
- ✓ 1 cup ACV

Inhale the steam produced to open airways and promote better breathing.

To produce a soothing tub soak, combine:
- ✓ A tub filled with hot water
- ✓ 3 cups ACV

Soak for 30 minutes. This technique can remove toxins from your body while also producing vapors which may help alleviate asthma symptoms.

Reduce Swelling

While most cases of swelling occur due to injuries or trauma, additionally, it may be derived from an unhealthy diet or displaced pressure. Nevertheless, the swelling started, so long as serious injuries like fractures and tendon or ligament damage are eliminated, you may effectively alleviate swelling safely and within the comfortable surroundings of your own home with apple cider vinegar treatments!

Apple cider vinegar may be used to treat swelling by:

- Contributing essential vitamins, minerals, enzymes, and acids to detoxifying your body.
- Replenishing essential stores of nutrients.
- Improving circulation and blood circulation for the affected area.
- Repairing damaged tissues

To produce a drink, combine:
- ✓ 1 cup of water
- ✓ 2 tablespoons of aloe vera juice
- ✓ 1 tablespoon of ACV

Drink daily to lessen swelling preventing further injury due to inflammation.

To produce a soak that may relieve swelling by drawing toxins from the body, improving circulation, and assisting in nutrient delivery towards the affected region, combine:
- ✓ A tub filled with tepid to warm water
- ✓ 2-4 cups of ACV

Soak for 30-45 minutes, allowing the ACV mixture to penetrate the affected area and address it from The within out.

To produce a spot treatment, soak a washcloth with:
- ✓ 1 cup ACV
- ✓ ½ cup of water

Sit using the swollen region elevated, and drape the washcloth on the affected area for thirty minutes at the same time every hour before swelling subsides.

Whitening of Teeth

Countless commercials on television, in magazines, and online continuously remind us our teeth ought to be whiter. One quick visit to the drugstore to get a teeth-whitening kit can simply become an excruciatingly lengthy tour from the multitude of products available in the market that promise "tangible results" in weeks, days, as well as short as you hour. These can cost from several dollars to higher than a hundred, not forgetting the teeth-whitening services provided by dentists that may cost thousands and take up plenty of time.

As well as the hits for your wallet as well as your schedule, the chemicals within these teeth-whitening products can leave you with susceptible teeth that are influenced by hot and cold foods and drinks, as well as breathing through the mouth area! Just forget about those treatments and instead consider apple cider vinegar for any teeth whitener that's inexpensive, natural, and quick. With powerful acids and enzymes that can effectively remove stains, kill germs, and promote a sufficient pH balance in the mouth, apple cider vinegar is used to boost the fitness of one's teeth, gums, and tongue, nonetheless it could also be used to whiten and brighten teeth.

An important note: Only use ACV like a whitening agent in its diluted form, safeguarding the enamel on your teeth from being stripped away.

To create an ACV teeth-whitening system, combine:
- ✓ ½ cup of ACV
- ✓ ½ cup of hot water

Swish and spit a mouthful in the mixture to prep your teeth for whitening.

Next, soak your toothbrush inside the mixture and brush your teeth daily as you'll typically, ensure to cover every area of one's teeth.

Finally, brush together with your regular toothpaste as you'll routinely.

Performing this routine daily will yield tangible results in just a matter of a couple of days to some weeks without unwanted adverse effects.

Resolves renal issues

The kidneys and bladder play important parts in ridding your body of toxins and bacteria. Spending so much time to flush the body's systems of waste material that are derived from every chemical result of your body (which you will find millions every minute, hour, and day!), the kidneys and bladder possess a whole lot of responsibility in safeguarding your wellbeing. When these powerhouse organs are compromised for some reason, the damaging effects on one's health could be overwhelming, affecting every system's function.

Many simple changes in lifestyle might help protect the fitness of your kidneys and bladder:
Drink sufficient water, eat a diet abundant with nutritious whole foods. Avoid harmful lifestyle habits like smoking and drinking excessively.

Exercise Daily

These actions will raise the functioning of the metabolism, improve blood quality and blood circulation, better detoxify your body, and improve immunity, which directly affects the kidney and bladder by minimizing the task positioned on them. ACV promotes the correct functioning of the organs by delivering nutrients, acids, and enzymes that:

Neutralize harmful stomach acids

Provide fibre for improved digestion

Maintain a sufficient balance of helpful bacteria that safeguard the fitness of the digestive and urinary systems

To produce a daily drink, combine:
- ✓ 1 cup of water
- ✓ 1 tablespoon of ACV

Drink daily.

To produce an ACV soak, combine:

Tub of tepid to warm water
- ✓ 2 cups ACV

Soak yourself in the perfect solution for thirty minutes once weekly.

Delivering protective nutrients towards the urinary tract while also detoxifying your body, these soaks can help prevent organisms from adversely affecting the fitness of the kidneys and bladder.

Chapter 6
Honey & Apple Cider Vinegar

Why do people mix apple cider vinegar and honey?

Vinegar could be created from most resources of fermentable carbs. Apple cider vinegar starts with apple juice being a base, that is then fermented twice with yeast. Its main ingredient is acetic acid, giving it its characteristically sour flavor.

Alternatively, honey is a sweet and viscous substance made by bees and stored inside a cluster of waxy, hexagonal cells referred to as a *honeycomb. Honey is an assortment of two sugars - fructose and glucose - with trace levels of pollen, micronutrients, and antioxidants.*

Many consider apple cider vinegar and honey to be always a tasty combination, as the sweetness of honey helps mellow Vinegar's puckery taste.

Consuming this tonic is considered to provide many health advantages. However, considering that both ingredients have already been studied separately, the consequences of the mixture specifically are largely unknown.

Apple cider vinegar and honey are consumed both individually and as a combination in natural medicine. Nevertheless, few studies have investigated the health effects of combining them.

Potential Benefits of ACV & Honey

Some individuals mix apple cider vinegar and honey because of its purported health advantages.

Acetic acid promote weight-loss

The acetic acid in apple cider vinegar continues to be studied like a weight reduction aid.

In a 12-week analysis in 144 adults with obesity, those ingesting 2 tablespoons (30ml) of apple cider vinegar diluted inside a 17-ounce (500-ml) drink daily experienced probably the most weight reduction and a 0.9% decrease in body fat, weighed against two control groups. Apple cider vinegar, also, has been shown to maintain you feel fuller longer since it decreases how quickly nutrients from foods are absorbed into the bloodstream - an impact that could further aid weight loss.

Still, whenever you combine honey and Vinegar, take into account that honey is saturated in calories and sugar and really should be consumed in moderation.

Help alleviate seasonal allergies and cold symptoms

Both honey and apple cider vinegar are believed natural antimicrobials. Honey is considered to help relieve seasonal allergies since it contains trace levels of pollen and plant compounds. Some studies also show that it could help relieve symptoms of allergic rhinitis, or hay fever.

Yet, it's unclear how adding apple cider vinegar to honey may influence these effects. Also, the mixture can help alleviate specific cold symptoms, such as coughing. What's more, because of its fermentation process, apple cider vinegar contains *probiotics*. These helpful bacteria aid digestion and boost immunity, which might assist you to fight a cold.

Improves heart health

The chlorogenic acid in Vinegar is considered to help decrease LDL cholesterol levels, potentially cutting your risk of cardiovascular disease. Plus, in rodent studies, honey has been shown to lessen high blood pressure, another risk factor for cardiovascular disease.

Also, it contains polyphenol antioxidants, which reduces cardiovascular disease risk by improving blood flow and preventing blood clots plus the oxidation of LDL cholesterol. Still, more research in this field is necessary. Furthermore, apple cider vinegar reduces inflammation and reduces your threat of plaque build-up within your arteries, which may protect heart health. Though more human studies have needed to explore this possible benefit. The potential health advantages of honey and apple cider Vinegar have mostly been studied separately. Vinegar is thought to aid weight-loss, while both are thought to improve heart health insurance and alleviate cold and seasonal allergic reactions.

Potential downside

While the health advantages of apple cider vinegar and honey have already been studied individually, hardly any is well known about the consequences of consuming them as a combination.

Possible effects on blood sugar levels and cholesterol

One report that examined an identical mixture containing namely grape vinegar and honey observed some adverse health effects. Within the 4-week learn, participants, drinking 8.5 ounces (250 ml) of water with 4 teaspoons (22 ml) of any grape-vinegar-and-honey mix plus some mint for flavor daily experienced slightly increased resistance to insulin, a hormone that regulates blood sugar. Increased insulin resistance is associated with type 2 diabetes.

Additionally, degrees of heart-protective HDL (very good) cholesterol decreased by the end of the analysis. Low HDL (bad) cholesterol is a risk factor for cardiovascular disease.

Take into account that it was a little and short-term study. More research is required to confirm these findings. A report investigating the consequences of honey and apple cider vinegar - instead of grape vinegar - is warranted.

Could be harsh on your stomach and teeth

The acidity of apple cider vinegar may worsen gastric reflux, while some people have claimed it improved their symptoms. However, considering that no substantial evidence can settle this debate, pay attention to your body's cues. Furthermore, because of its acidity, apple cider vinegar has been proven to erode tooth enamel, potentially upping your threat of tooth decay.

Consequently, it's recommended to dilute the Vinegar with filtered water and rinse the mouth area with only water after drinking it. More research is required to determine the consequences of combining it with honey. Interestingly, some studies show honey might help defend against *gingivitis, cavities, and bad breath.*

Can be saturated in sugar

Depending on just how much honey you add, your mixture is quite saturated in sugar. It's vital that you limit added sugars in what you eat, as consuming an excessive amount of it can have unwanted effects on your general health. An excessive amount of added sugar - especially from sweetened beverages - is associated with an increased threat of conditions like cardiovascular disease and obesity.

Though smaller amounts of honey can match a healthy diet plan and may offer health advantages, it's vital that you appreciate it in moderation. Drinking apple cider vinegar and honey may have downsides, including unwanted effects for tooth and stomach health. More research is necessary on the medical effects and risks of the mixture.

Purported effects on body alkalinity

The pH scale ranges from 0 to 14, or from most acidic to more alkalines. Some people declare that eating particular foods or supplements, such as apple cider vinegar and honey, could make your body even more alkaline and prevent diseases like cancer and osteoporosis.

However, the body features complex systems set up to keep your blood pH level between 7.35 and 7.45, which is necessary because of its proper functioning. In case your blood pH falls beyond this range, the results could be fatal. Foods and supplements, including an assortment of apple cider vinegar and honey, do little to influence blood alkalinity. Food just affects the pH degree of your urine. Whether apple cider vinegar can transform your body's acid-base balance, in the long run, have to be investigated. Some people declare that apple cider vinegar might help alkalize the body and defend against disease. However, the body carefully regulates its blood pH levels, and foods and supplements only affect the pH of the urine.

Best Uses of ACV

In natural medicine, 1 tablespoon (15ml) of apple cider vinegar and 2 teaspoons (21grams) of honey is diluted in 8 ounces (240 ml) of warm water and enjoyed like a soothing tonic before bedtime or upon waking. You can enjoy this warm mixture alone or add lemon, ginger, fresh mint, cayenne pepper, or ground cinnamon for flavor. *When you have gastric reflux or heartburn, it's better to drink it one hour before you lay down to diminish symptoms.*

Moreover, apple cider vinegar and honey are complementary ingredients within a culinary context. Together, they can make an excellent base for salad dressings, marinades, and brines for pickling vegetables. However, the safety of combining apple cider vinegar and honey for small children is not studied. You need to speak with your son or daughter's pediatrician before using this mixture being a home remedy.

Additionally, *children younger than 12 months of age shouldn't eat honey and apple cider vinegar because of the threat of botulism, a rare and potentially fatal illness due to bacteria.* Apple cider vinegar and honey could be used widely in people older than one. To drink it like a hot tonic, dilute the mix in tepid to warm water before bedtime or upon waking. It is also used in your kitchen to dress salads, marinate meats, and pickled vegetables.

Apple cider vinegar and honey tend to be combined in natural medicine.

The mixture is normally diluted in hot water and drunk before bedtime or upon rising. It's claimed to assist weight reduction and improve seasonal allergies and blood pressure. Still, most research targets the effects of every ingredient separately. Without much been known about the tremendous medical effects of this mixture, it's instead a delicious and comforting drink to relish at the beginning or end of your respective day.

Chapter 7
Apple Cider Vinegar for Hair Care

Do you spend a lot of time and dollars on your regular hair regimen?

Do you find yourself coping with unruly locks that lack the quantity, shine, or length you imagine?

Are you currently finding it harder to keep up your hair's natural splendor?

Or are you just sick and tired of wasting money on chemical-laden hair-care products that promise the entire world but neglect to deliver?

If you consider just how many hair products you regularly utilize, between shampooing and styling, imaginable just how much residue from those products gets left out.

All that residue and build-up from the merchandise that is intended to support hair effectively actually hinder natural growth, shine, body, highlights, and a lot more! Due to the damage that this build-up could cause for your hair's follicles, cuticles, pores, and ends, you will be left with unmanageable tresses that are so unhealthy, and no product may help!

Search no further: *apple cider vinegar will restore natural health in your hair and assist you to attain the hair you've always imagined!* ACV contains a fantastic selection of naturally occurring acids, enzymes, vitamins, and minerals that work synergistically to provide the nourishment required by healthy hair. These constituents may be found in different formulations with functional capabilities ranging from a clarifying rinse and shampoo to a highly effective preparation to get more vibrant and longer-lasting color treatments, and it is secure enough to drink.

Supported with scientific explanations of how and just why this product, as well as the combinations and treatments for every specific benefit work to remove the hair issues you cope with daily, these *easy-to-create* and *simple-to-use treatments*, can easily supply the results you want while repairing the damage that beautiful hair "care" products did.

The end result is this: If you wish to achieve the results you might have dreamt of for a long time, sick and tired of spending on products and treatments that aren't delivering, and want to use an all-natural product, try apple cider vinegar. Start repairing flowing hair and get on the right path to the stunning hair you imagine by implementing these ACV treatments today!

Help Hair Thinning

Thinning hair is an embarrassing condition, and it doesn't only strike older men. Women of most ages have become a significant area of the consumer pool, searching for remedies to avoid hair thinning. While prescription medications and over-the-counter medications promise to provide robust results, they often contain severe chemicals and additives that may pose health threats and aggravate certain medical ailments.

If you're seeking to reap the advantages of hair thinning treatments safely and effectively with essential natural products, search no further when compared to a trusty bottle of apple cider vinegar. Through the use of apple cider vinegar right to the solution to hair thinning, you can:
- *Improve the blood flow from the scalp.*
- *Enhance the blood circulation to hair roots.*

- *Ensure the effective delivery of essential nutrients towards the scalp.*

These health-boosting benefits supplied by ACV help promote hair regrowth and prevent hair thinning. ACV also includes valuable vitamins, minerals, and proteins, offering your skin with essential nutrients needed to produce healthy hair and keep maintaining quality proteins inside the hair shaft.

To Produce a Hair Tonic, Combine:

- ✓ 2 tablespoons ACV.
- ✓ 1 tablespoon water.
- ✓ 1/2 teaspoon cayenne pepper.

Apply right to the source of hair thinning, rubbing the mixture into the scalp for five minutes. Let it take a seat on the scalp for one hour before shampooing as usual. You can begin to find out results within 2-4 weeks.

Two chemical substances in cayenne, *capsaicin, and quercetin,* will be the beneficial components that help stimulate hair regrowth by stimulating hair roots and improving blood circulation in the scalp.

Make Your Hair Rinse

Some hair-care products effectively provide what they promise, and many leave unsightly residue and build-up around the hair roots, hair shafts, and scalp. This build-up can result in excessively oily hair, unmanageable frizz, or lackluster color. Comically, many hair products promise to eliminate this residue through the use of chemicals and harsh abrasives that may result in hair that's dry and unmanageable, meaning you traded one problem for another.

Through the use of apple cider vinegar like a rinse, following a regular shampooing and conditioning treatments, you can effectively remove residue and restore your hair's health, shine, and color naturally and without unwanted adverse effects. With acids and enzymes that cleanse and minerals and vitamins that nourish, apple cider vinegar can clear the hair of debris and build-up without damaging the hair's follicles or disrupting the scalp's pH balance.

To Produce a Hair Rinse, Combine:
- ✓ 1 cup of water,

- ✓ 1/2 cup of ACV.

Apply it to the hair following your routine of shampooing and conditioning. Permit the mixture to take a seat on the hair and scalp for five minutes before rinsing with tepid to warm water. Repeating this process with almost every other wash will make sure your hair stays free from build-up that weighs down hair.

Produce Your Shampoo

Some shampoos leave you with luscious locks that bounce, shine, and stay frizz-free, while some leave hair feeling weighed down, dry out, or filled with frizz. Checking out different brands could be costly, time-consuming, and damaging for your hair. Through the use of apple cider vinegar being a shampoo alternative, you may naturally cleanse the hair and add beauty and health in your strands. You may even discover and feel a noticeable difference in the grade of beautiful hair after just one single treatment!

ACV is inexpensive, natural, and doesn't contain harsh chemicals and additions (that would raise the frequency of bad hair days).

ACV will give flowing hair with these excellent benefits:
- Cleanse hair of grime and build-up.
- Add health-fortifying minerals and vitamins right to the hair and scalp for improved shine, volume, and bounce.
- Provide from therapeutic proteins to pH-neutralizing enzymes.
- Promote hair health insurance and restore beauty to strands.
- Gently remove environmental deposits.

To Create Shampoo, Combine inside a bottle:
- ✓ 1/2 cup of ACV
- ✓ 2 tablespoons of lemon juice
- ✓ 1 cup of water

Utilize the mixture instead of your shampoo, massaging it into the scalp and strands, rinsing, and proceeding to condition while you routinely would.

You should use this shampoo substitute every wash, or utilize it alternately together with your regular shampoo.

Produce Your Conditioner

Nowadays, you'll find deep conditioning treatments in the home and in the salon, as well as balms and solutions that promise to leave hair silky and hydrated. All of the conditioning treatments are dizzying. Dependant on whether the hair is usually oily, dry, curly, or straight, different conditioners made to treat all hair types may fall flat on delivering their promised results.

Surprisingly enough, precisely the same bottle of apple cider vinegar you utilize for your regular tonics that keeps you healthy and energized. It may also work wonders like a conditioner for hair of most types, shades, and textures. Several treatment options could be obtainable, but few supply the nutrients within ACV, and are as inexpensive as ACV, and offer results following the initial treatment as ACV does! Combined with additional conditioning the different parts of coconut oil, *ACV is an efficient conditioner that tames frizz, fights tangles, and keeps locks lustrous while improving the pH degrees of the scalp and closing the hair roots.*

To Produce a Conditioner, Combine in a bottle:
- ✓ 1/2 cup of ACV
- ✓ 1/2 cup of liquid coconut oil
- ✓ 1 cup of water

Apply the procedure to your hair, cover the hair using a shower cap, and wait for thirty minutes. Then rinse and dry, revealing renewed hair with restored health.

Combat Baldness

Baldness may appear due to genetics, repeated damaging hair treatments, or insufficient dietary elements that support the healthy growth of hair.

In its unfiltered state, ACV contains several helpful enzymes, proteins, vitamins, minerals, and naturally occurring acids that combine to:

- Contribute cleansing and restorative elements right to the source of baldness.
- Remove agitating causes that may contribute to baldness. Enhance the conditions with the hair and

scalp, promoting fresh hair regrowth and maintaining the fitness of that hair regrowth.

Chemical-laden hair-regenerating products can irritate the scalp, damage the hair, and hinder the absorption and usage of essential elements necessary for healthy hair regrowth. Instead, only use natural ingredient shampoos, conditioners, and treatments such as ACV.

Finally, to spot-treat baldness and internally balance essential physical nutrients, you should use two effective treatments: *a topical ACV treatment and an ingested ACV tonic.*

To produce a tonic, combine:
- ✓ 1/2 cup of water
- ✓ 1/2 cup of ACV
- ✓ 1/2 teaspoon of cayenne pepper.

Apply the mixture right to the scalp in the areas where baldness is appearing. Leave the mixture within the scalp for an interval of thirty minutes, then wash with shampoo and apply conditioner after that as normal. Third, repeat the procedure regularly has shown to boost baldness in 2-4 weeks!

To Produce a drinkable tonic, combine:
- ✓ 1 cup of water
- ✓ 1 tablespoon of ACV

Mix and drink daily.

This solution supplies the dietary components in ACV like the vitamins, minerals, enzymes, and acids that:

- Support the fitness of systems directly linked to the growth and health of hair, such as metabolism and blood circulation.
- Resolve deficiencies that may contribute to baldness, such as some B vitamins, vitamin C, vitamin D, and iron.

Detangle Hair

Whenever your hair is a tangled mess, and you have trouble simply brushing or combing it after a shower, you might be inclined to employ a detangling product. Even though many products available on the market promise to leave beautiful hair healthy and free from tangles, a lot of them contain chemicals or unnatural chemicals that may strip healthy elements from hair, leaving your strands lackluster and damaged. To fight tangles while keeping the fitness of hair, try ACV! Having in it restorative and essential minerals and vitamins, ACV can reduce tangles by detaching residue and build-up left out from cleaning products, while also moisturizing and conditioning your strands and making them more manageable and better to style.

To Produce a Detangling Spray, Combine inside a spray bottle:
- ✓ 1/2 cup of ACV
- ✓ 1 cup of water

Spray flowing hair using the ACV solution from your scalp towards the ends of the hair, combing through locks and relieving tangles.

Reduce Frizz

Frizzy hair is a frustrating condition that may be caused by the elements or extensive contact with damaging elements within hair products and hair treatments. The crux of curly hair issues is high porosity, which is due to the shaft of hair strands remaining open and struggling to retain moisture. The blow-drying of the strands makes them vulnerable to the effects of the climate or styling products and treatments that result in hair appearing "frizzy."

By delivering naturally therapeutic proteins and nutrients in your hair strands, it is possible to spot-treat frizziness and revels in healthy, shiny, manageable hair. You may find "natural" products available in the market, but make sure to browse the ingredients carefully, many are labeled *"natural"* however they nonetheless contain particular preservatives or synthetic materials that may result in hair damage. To avoid unnecessary "bad hair days" due to frizz, you will need to search no further than apple cider vinegar. ACV contains rich levels of proteins and enzymes, offering hair with restorative health advantages.

To create an in-shower anti-frizz treatment, combine within a bottle:

- ✓ 1/2cup of ACV
- ✓ 1/2 cup of water
- ✓ 2 teaspoons of liquid coconut oil.

After conditioning within the shower, apply the mixture to your hair and leave it on for five minutes. Then rinse the solution through the hair and dry as you'll routinely.

To Produce a Prestyling, Frizz-Fighting Solution, Combine inside a Spray bottle:

- ✓ 1 cup of water
- ✓ 1/2 cup of ACV.

Saturate damp hair using the ACV spray. After allowing the spray to stay for five minutes, towel-dry and style as you'll routinely.

Prevent Split Ends

Split ends occur when the end of the hair strand breaks into two strands that, when checked out, split the hair from underneath up. Not merely does this damage the hair; nonetheless, it could make the appearance plus the maintenance and styling of hair difficult and frustrating.

By trimming only the ends of your respective hair monthly, you could prevent split ends before they start and keep healthy hair free from split-end damage. Yet another way to avoid split ends is usually to make sure that you have the correct intake of essential minerals and vitamins that contribute to healthy hair regrowth, like *silica, calcium, vitamin C, and B vitamins.*

A plentiful vitamin and mineral intake will improve your hair's health from the within out and stop split ends from occurring. To take care of split ends most effectively, you should use all-natural, unfiltered, organic apple cider vinegar as an ingested preventive measure and a topical treatment, providing rest from split ends forever!

To Produce a solution that ensures your vitamin and mineral intake is optimal, combine;

- ✓ 1 cup of water
- ✓ 1 tablespoon of ACV

Drink daily.

To produce a localized treatment for split ends, combine;

- ✓ 1/2 cup water
- ✓ 1/2 cup ACV
- ✓ 1/4 cup mashed avocado.

Rub the mixture into the bottom 1/4 of hair, and make to set for thirty minutes before rinsing thoroughly. Continue doing this treatment several times weekly, and you may effectively prevent split ends, seeing results in just a matter of several short weeks.

Kill and Stop Headlice

Head lice is a frustrating and challenging issue, primarily because the most affected population is school-aged children. In close quarters like classrooms with many children, head lice are often transferred from individual to individual. Limiting Contact with anyone with verified head lice may be the first preventive measure that may effectively decrease the potential for contracting head lice. When you are coping with a verified case of head lice, though, you mustn't only treat the top lice, but also take protective measures to guarantee the lice die and also have no potential for time to cause the problem again. Many drugstore products can be found that may treat head lice. However, most contain chemicals and synthetic additives that may be hazardous to your wellbeing or dangerous to adults and children with specific skin sensitivities. *As an all-natural alternative, try ACV.*

To produce a head lice treatment:
Apply undiluted apple cider vinegar to the hair and scalp, within the hair with a shower cap. Let the Vinegar stay on the hair for at least 4-5 hours. After removing the cap and rinsing the hair with water, carefully comb through the hair with a fine-tooth comb, removing the nits and eggs. Repeat this procedure daily until all lice and eggs have died.

Promote Hair Regrowth

The amount of hair-growth products available in the market is overwhelmingly large and is also increasing each year. The difference between one product and another could be the chemical components, the claims to be "all-natural," or the guarantees that growth will follow the product's use. While the promotions can seem promising, the actual results can vary product to product and person to person depending on several factors. By combining a number of effective hair-growth methods with ACV, you can effectively and inexpensively improve your hair growth naturally. Apple cider vinegar has long been promoted for a large number of uses that promote health because of its high amounts of essential vitamins and minerals. With natural acids, enzymes, and proteins also contained within every drop of ACV; it is now accepted as an effective ingredient for treating hair loss and supporting hair growth. By massaging the scalp daily, eating a balanced diet high in protein, and minimizing the hair's exposure to heat treatments and harmful chemicals, you can maintain hair health.

To produce a nightly hair regrowth treatment, combine:
- ✓ 1 cup of ACV
- ✓ 1 cup of aloe vera juice.

Apply right to the scalp and through the entire hair towards the ends, cover using a shower cap, and sleep using the applied mixture to the hair for 7-8 hours. Shower or rinse the hair each day. You can enhance the health of your hair, restore natural essential nutrients, and see and feel the results in 2-4 weeks.

Remove Hard Water Residue

The word *"hard water"* is used to spell out water containing minerals from rocks and sediments in the region from which water was obtained, in the procedure for the water, or between treatment as well as your home. When you are coping with discolored, foul-smelling, or hard-to-manage hair that doesn't suds up when you shampoo, hard water could be to blame.

The simplest way to improve hard water is to install a treatment pump or filter that can remove the minerals of your water. However, these can be expensive and sometimes ineffective. Regardless of your long-term plan to treat your water, it is essential to treat your hair to rid it of the hard water effects as quickly as possible. Over-the-counter treatments for hard water hair can be costly or loaded with chemicals, so opting for a natural treatment like ACV may be your safest and most effective way to achieve your healthy hair again. With acids and enzymes galore, apple cider vinegar is one of the safest and most effective treatments for ridding hair of residue and build-up. When it comes to removing mineral build-up, ACV is just as effective as top-of-the-line products but can do so quickly, safely, and without posing a risk to hair or skin health.

Packed with nourishing nutrients that also help to restore essential vitamins and minerals directly into your strands' cuticles, pores, and shafts, apple cider vinegar can also help reverse damage done by mineral deposits on the hair.

What's the best part?

The power of ACV's enzymes and acids can remove deposits on hair.

To produce a hair rinse, combine:
- ✓ 1 cup of ACV
- ✓ 1 cup of water

Apply the perfect solution to hair following shampooing and conditioning as usual. Permit the solution to stay on hair for five minutes before rinsing.

You can even utilize the shampoo and conditioner recipes explained in this book for natural alternatives to shampoos and conditioners that may leave residues behind.

Add Shine

Probably one of the most common complaints about hair is that it's dull, and haircare companies know this all too well. To the rescue of lackluster hair, an incredible number of products that promise to bring back the light-reflective shine to your dull mane are available at your favorite grocery store, drugstore, salon, or hair product source and can range in price from $1 to over $100!

If you're hoping to remedy your lackluster locks and return the beautiful glow we associate with healthy hair, you needn't look any further than your trusty bottle of apple cider vinegar.

By introducing apple cider vinegar into your diet and hair treatment routine, you can:

- Restore the natural balance of nutrients in your body's systems that promote hair health, thereby topically increasing your hair's condition and an appearance by stripping away residue and build-up left out from styling products.
- Repair damage that was done by heat and chemical treatments intended to style, color, or treat hair.

To produce a shiny-hair solution, combine:
- ✓ 1 cup of water

- ✓ 1 tablespoon ACV

Drink daily to provide the right amount of vitamins, minerals, acids, and enzymes that help out with maintaining hair health.

To produce a topical hair solution, combine:
- ✓ 1 cup of water
- ✓ 1 cup of ACV
- ✓ 2 tablespoons of gas of peppermint

After shampooing and conditioning, apply the solution to hair and sort out strands. Permit the mixture to stay for 5-10 minutes before rinsing thoroughly.

This treatment can restore hair health for the shaft, pores, and cuticles of hair strands, assisting in repairing damage and restoring a wholesome sheen naturally.

Highlight Hair

If you're trying to find natural at-home solutions to highlight flowing hair that can substitute your expensive and hair-damaging salon highlight treatments, it is possible to exchange the costly chemical treatments for all-natural ACV to attain the same beautiful results. ACV contains several acids and enzymes that will help naturally lighten hair strands when subjected to sunlight. You just have to combine ACV with other things that assist in the lightening process while also conditioning the treated strands with natural oils.

To produce a hair lightener, combine at room temperature:
- ✓ 1 cup of water
- ✓ 1/2 cup of fresh-squeezed lemon juice
- ✓ 1/2 cup of liquid coconut oil
- ✓ 1/2cup of ACV

Apply it on the hair, and invite the wet hair to come in contact with sunlight for 20-30 minutes. This treatment can enhance the appearance of highlights naturally, inexpensively, and effectively in less than one treatment.

Drive Back Chlorine Damage

If you've ever seen a pool-loving child during the warm months, you've seen the chlorine after-effects that may transform the color of any locks to some dark green, dry the hair, and turn even the most amazing tresses to one of unmanageable frizz and damaged split ends.

If you can't resist the pool and can't bear the very thought of chlorine damage, what's the protective treatment which you can use?

What treatment option can reverse chlorine damage as well as prevent it?

What treatment option is inexpensive, requires no visits to the salon, and may be utilized daily without damaging hair? **Apple cider vinegar.**

With natural compounds that close the hair shaft correctly, protecting the hair strands from chemical damage such as chlorine damage, apple cider vinegar creates an ideal environment for hair to block infiltrating chemicals that may destroy hair quality from the inside out. Containing natural components that strip away grime, build-up, and excess chemical residue, apple cider vinegar can also be used as an effective rinse that can rid even the blondest of hair of the green chlorine sheen.

To produce a chlorine-busting rinse, combine within a spray bottle:

- ✓ 1 cup of water
- ✓ 2 cups of ACV.

Apply the mixture before and after exposing hair to chlorine by saturating the hair with the perfect solution and shampoo and then rinse it as you will routinely.

Promote Scalp Health

ACV is an option to expensive, synthetic products that could or might not work to make your scalp healthier. It's an instant and inexpensive, all-natural, nutrient-rich option, whether your issue with scalp health is mild or severe. The fitness of your scalp directly affects the grade of your entire day. If that sounds a little extreme, talk with someone who is suffering from severe dandruff, bouts of baldness or hair thinning, or frequent itchy scalp, and you'll discover that scalp health is a serious business. By walking into any hair-care aisle of nearly every store, you can see that scalp health can be a lucrative business, with a large number of products made to restore health for your scalp at a cost. Whether you pay out that price in the trouble of the merchandise, or by experiencing health conditions that may be aggravated or the result of the chemicals or synthetic ingredients within the product, lots of the scalp-restorative products don't surpass their promises or are more than you bargained.

To revive health for your scalp, combine:
- ✓ 1 cup of water
- ✓ 1/2 cup of ACV
- ✓ 1 teaspoon of cayenne pepper
- ✓ 1 teaspoon of organic honey.

Wet hair and apply the mixture to the scalp, rubbing into the scalp thoroughly. Allow mixture to stay on hair and scalp for thirty minutes before rinsing, shampooing, and conditioning as usual. Repeat daily or weekly.

Remove Product Residue

Do you use shampoo, conditioner, straightening products, keratin products, curling agents, gel, hairspray, mousse, or leave-in conditioner, or have regular treatments in your hair designed to color or style your locks? If you're among the vast amounts of consumers who answered yes, you almost certainly possess considerable product residue on your hair. When you may not see by simply taking a look at or touching hair, the styling products and treatments you utilize to cleanse, condition, or treat beautiful hair can leave behind a film of chemical build-up or residue even after washing.

If you're among the thousands of people who use clarifying products that promise to rid the flowing hair of the unhealthy build-up, you might be surprised to discover that many of them just partially solve the issue, and many can leave behind additional residue. Consider ACV to seriously cleanse hair without harsh chemicals or additives that may strip nutrients along with build-up. Clarifying enzymes and acids that naturally occur in apple cider vinegar will be the compelling contents that make it a clarifying effective product, yet safe. With this suggested treatment of two different applications of ACV for your hair, you can easily take away the build-up of residue left out by hair products and follow-up, which has a therapeutic nutrient-rich application that may leave your hair healthier than ever before.

To produce a soak, combine:
- ✓ 1 cup of ACV
- ✓ 1/2 cup of water.

Soak hair from scalp to end with the perfect solution and encompass hair having a shower cap, allowing the mixture to stay on your hair for thirty minutes. Rinsing with only water, you can shower as usual, but apply no product on the hair.

To produce a nourishing conditioner, combine:
- ✓ 1 cup of ACV
- ✓ ½ cup of liquid coconut oil
- ✓ ½ cup of water.

Two hours after rinsing the ACV soak from your scalp, apply this mixture right to the hair and scalp, massaging it in. Permit the solution to stay on hair for thirty minutes, then rinse the solution with normal water. Comb and towel-dry.

Chapter 8
Apple Cider Vinegar for Skin Care

A vast number of women all over the world assist in contributing to the multibillion-dollar industry that targets skincare. Each day, we see countless messages that remind us in our wrinkles, blemishes, redness, liver spots, and varicose veins questionnaire, combined with the message that people could be proactive in reversing aging and improving their beauty simply by paying a few dollars here and some even more dollars there on products made to support us declare victory over the war of skin conditions which make it less appealing. *Before spending another penny on the most recent and most exceptional skin-care product, read this phenomenal portion of apple cider vinegar's uses for skincare.*

Inexpensive, all-natural, organic apple cider vinegar is used to correct and restore the fitness of skin, which this chapter is focused on the countless applications you can merely and very quickly implement starting today to renew your skin layer and experience better about yourself effectively. Without chemicals, additives, or synthetic materials, apple cider vinegar would help you achieve true lasting beauty within the comfortable surroundings of your own home, replacing the expensive chemical-laden alternatives that may wreak havoc on your skin and do more harm than sound.

The best part of apple cider vinegar is what it could supply to your skin layer with regards to nourishment. Packed with vitamins that become powerful antioxidants, ACV can repair skin surface damage and provide antioxidants which assist in preventing further damage due to unhealthy changes within skin cells. Minerals that promotes adequate blood circulation and improved circulation will also be vital to your skin's health insurance and beautiful appearance, making apple cider vinegar a lot more appealing. Naturally occurring enzymes and acids that combine to maintain skin clear and clean without harsh unwanted effects is just yet another good thing about this natural ingredient.

Cleanse Your Pores

That person is subjected to several toxins during the day. Airborne elements and visible dirt and grime adversely affect the looks and health of your skin. While environmental factors are to blame to an extent, the more common contributor to clogged pores is touching your face with your hands, which you likely do dozens of times per day, consciously or subconsciously. When your pores become clogged with unhealthy deposits from your hands, the skin is unable to "breathe," and it can develop an oily, greasy, or excessively dry condition.

Many cleansers on the market contain harsh or abrasive components that can aggravate the skin's natural balance of oils and pH, and lead to unhealthy or uncomfortable skin conditions. As a natural alternative to chemical-laden products, *apple cider vinegar provides cleansing properties that rid the skin of harmful deposits and keep the skin's pores open and healthy.* By restoring the natural pH balance of the skin, ACV has also shown to regulate the oils produced by the skin, resulting in a healthier balance of oil production and minimizing the clogging of pores.

To produce a pore cleanser, combine within a bowl:
- ✓ ½ cup of tepid to warm water
- ✓ ½ cup of ACV

Make use of a facecloth to soak up the liquid, ring out the surplus, and gently rub your skin using the towel. Repeatedly rinse and reabsorb the ACV mixture, reapplying the mixture for the skin until the skin looks and feels refreshed and clear.

Tone Your Skin Layer

If you're among the many individuals who spend a fair penny on top-of-the-line skin toners, instead use apple cider vinegar! With regards to skin treatments, the same elements that produce ACV effective in treating general health conditions make it a fantastic product for treating conditions of your skin as well. The goal of a skin toner is to eliminate dead skin cells and oil, refreshing the region of the facial skin and revealing a rejuvenated layer of skin that appears clean, clear, and supple.

ACV's vitamins and naturally occurring acids certainly are a safe and effective way to improve the look and feel of skin while also restoring the natural balance of oils and pH of the skin. Specifically, the acetic and malic acids contained within apple cider vinegar improve the health and appearance of the skin by:

- Softly removing dead skin cells,
- Balancing the pH degrees of your skin,
- Removing dirt and oils from your pores,
- Treating the sources of acne and unsightly blemishes,
- Providing vitamin C-based antioxidant advantages to restore skin cell health insurance and reverse oxidative damage.

To produce a skin toner, combine:
- ✓ ½ cup of warm water
- ✓ ½ cup of ACV

Soak a cotton ball in the solution and apply right to your skin of the facial skin and neck. The rest of the mixture could be kept in the dark, cool place within an airtight container.

Minimize Psoriasis

Psoriasis can be an uncomfortable and unsightly condition that's regarded as due to trauma to your skin, stress, smoking, excessive alcohol consumption, sun exposure, and certain medications. Seen as a silvery or red patch of skin that could or might not itch, psoriasis is a non-contagious condition caused by the body's autoimmune system seeing your skin cells as pathogens and overstimulating the production of skin cells. Even though many over-the-counter creams can offer relief of psoriasis and/or treat your skin condition, many contain harsh chemicals or produce undesirable side effects that can further irritate the skin.

Lifestyle changes that minimize the factors that are assumed to contribute to the condition (such as quitting smoking and minimizing alcohol consumption, sun exposure, and stress) will help improve the effectiveness of any psoriasis treatment. Apple cider vinegar has become a notable treatment for skin conditions like psoriasis because of the multitude of beneficial elements it can provide internally, as well as to the site of irritation. ACV provides:

- Immunity-boosting vitamin C
- Blood-quality-improving enzymes
- Reparative antioxidant properties.

Apple cider vinegar is an all-natural product that may enhance the health of your skin layer while also maintaining proper functioning with the body's systems that directly support the skin's health.

To produce a localized treatment, combine:
- ✓ ½ cup of water
- ✓ ½ cup of ACV.

Soak a towel in the perfect solution is and use it right to the affected area for thirty minutes.

To produce a drink that supports overall skin health, combine:

- 1 cup of water
- 1 tablespoon of ACV

Drink daily.

Ease Sunburn

When your skin is subjected to excessive sunlight, with or without sunblock, the irritation that results isn't just uncomfortable and unsightly; nonetheless, it could be downright dangerous! Increasingly more research directly associates sun contact with unhealthy and even tumors of your skin cells. If you've got a sunburn, the simplest way to soothe and repair the skin is to apply natural restorative elements that aid in the regeneration and repair of the skin's cells.

One of the most effective agents in improving cell health is vitamin C, and many products in the market that claim to improve skin health contain this essential vitamin. While the cosmetic products available temporarily relieve sunburns or improve the look and feel of skin, few contain the combination of elements provided by apple cider vinegar that can improve skin health safely, naturally, and effectively. Through its healthy acids and enzymes that restore the natural balance of the naturally occurring oils produced by the skin, *ACV alleviates the tightening and burning sensations resulting from sunburn.* Replenishing the vitamin C stores on-site, topical use of ACV also aids in the cell regeneration in the skin while preventing free radical damage that can cause cancerous cell changes.

To produce a skin soak, combine:
- ✓ ½ cup of cold water
- ✓ ½ cup of ACV

Apply the ACV mixture right to the skin on the moist towel or sponge.

To produce a soothing soak, combine:
- ✓ A tub filled with water
- ✓ 2 cups of ACV

Soak for thirty minutes.

To produce a drink, combine:
- ✓ 1 cup water or freshly squeezed orange juice

- ✓ 1 tablespoon of aloe vera juice, organic
- ✓ 1 tablespoon of ACV

Take the solution 3x daily.

By combining these three treatments, you could alleviate the symptoms that emanated from sunburn and effectively treat cell damage that resulted from sunlight exposure.

Remove Acne

Acne sufferers have long sought out the resolution of blemishes that may appear on the facial skin, neck, chest, back, and arms. Prescribed drugs and over-the-counter treatments are occasionally expensive, ineffective, or packed with severe chemicals and additives. To be able to treat the problem safely, naturally, and effectively, acne sufferers may use apple cider vinegar in several ways. *Apple cider vinegar could be found in four effective treatment plans (as a soak, tonic, localized treatment, or facial mask) that are inexpensive, simple to use, and completely risk-free!* The treatments that include apple cider vinegar, when applied right to your skin in a soak/bath, facial cleanser, or mask, are intended to achieve a number of regulatory and restorative balances in the skin that will help to alleviate the causes of acne and prevent future occurrences. When applied directly to the skin, apple cider vinegar's antioxidants, vitamins, minerals, acids, and enzymes work synergistically to:

- Restore a standard pH to your skin
- Regulate oil production that may result in the clogging of pores
- Reduce inflammation in the site of blemishes
- Improve circulation inside the skin to reduce the appearance of blemishes and redness that so often accompany acne.

To produce a soak, combine:
- ✓ *A tub filled with water*
- ✓ *2-4 cups of ACV*

Soak for 30 minutes.

To produce a tonic, combine:
- ✓ *1 cup of water*
- ✓ *1 tablespoon of ACV*

Drink daily.

To produce a localized treatment, combine:
- ✓ ½ cup of ACV
- ✓ ½ cup of water

Apply on the skin as needed.

To produce a facial mask, combine:
- ✓ ½ mashed avocado
- ✓ ½ cup of ACV

Apply evenly to handle, allowing to create for ten minutes daily.

Diminish Eczema

Eczema is a persistent skin irritation seen as a red, rough, patchy regions of skin. Eczema shows to be frustrating by allergens, leading doctors to categorize the problem as an immune disorder. Since there is no known cure for eczema, there are numerous treatments available that are effective in reducing the frequency of the condition's appearance, as well as reducing the symptoms that derive from the uncomfortable condition. In case your eczema is the effect of a particular allergen, minimizing your contact with it will relieve the problem significantly.

While there are a variety of products available in the market made to calm the symptoms of eczema, apple cider vinegar is an all-natural remedy worth trying. Acting as an antibacterial, antifungal, and antiviral agent that also provides essential nutrients and hypoallergenic properties, ACV can reduce inflammation on-site, keep the irritated and inflamed part of eczema free from agitating environmental elements carefully, and also help soothe and repair the skin's cells suffering from the reaction.

To produce a localized treatment, combine equal parts:
- ✓ Water
- ✓ ACV

Soak a towel in the result and connect with the affected area for thirty minutes.

To produce a drink, combine:
- ✓ 1 cup of freshly juiced strawberries
- ✓ 1 tablespoon of ACV

Drink daily.

The vitamin C and acetic and malic acids combine to bolster a healthy disease fighting capability and reparation from the skin's cells.

Soothe Diaper Rash

The word *"diaper rash"* is mostly used to refer to the irritation on a baby's backside, caused by moist conditions that are ever-present in wet or soiled diapers. Precisely the same factors that contribute to diaper rash on the baby's bottom can occur in a grown-up of any age and result in the same uncomfortable condition. Adults will get "diaper rash" from:

- Debris left out after wiping the genitals and anus after using the toilet.
- Wearing tight-fitting clothes which make it problematic for the nether regions to "breathe" rendering it challenging to walk, sit, stand, or wear particular types of clothing, diaper rash can hinder the lifestyle of babies and adults alike.

Even though many creams and powders promise relief of the problem, ACV not merely soothes symptoms, but it additionally really helps to repair and restore the skin's health. Containing vitamins, minerals, and antioxidants that help out with the regeneration of skin cells, ACV also provides antiseptic, antibacterial, antifungal, and antiviral properties that help with keeping skin free from irritants and infection-causing stimuli.

To produce a localized treatment, combine:
- ✓ ½ cup of ACV
- ✓ ½ cup of water

Soak a cotton ball or soft towel in the perfect solution is and connect with the affected area gently every quarter-hour during the period of 2 hours.

Relieve Hemorrhoids

Hemorrhoids are mostly experienced by older people and women that are pregnant, but they may also strike women and men of most ages. Usually caused by pushing or straining the bowels while defecating, hemorrhoids are swollen veins that may be external or internal and can exist extremely unpleasant or just annoying. Sometimes associated with blood inside the stool, hemorrhoids are usually not cause for concern but can require surgery in severe cases. *The tips for treatment of hemorrhoids range between skin medications to ingested digestion aids that may combine to ease the problem by curing the reason and treating the resulting symptoms.*

If you're seeking natural alternatives towards the chemical-laden, over-the-counter choices that may cause diarrhea and constipation or further agitate the affected area, try apple cider vinegar. *Apple cider vinegar is used as a highly effective treatment for hemorrhoids, and it is reported to supply relief from the within out that far surpasses the over-the-counter alternatives.* Acting as digestive aids that facilitate moving out of waste with the digestive system better, *the pectin, acetic acid, and malic acid* within ACV combine to bind with waste and lubricate the stools because they go through the bowels, requiring less pressure on the bowels during defecation and reducing the incidence of hemorrhoids.

To produce a drink to alleviate hemorrhoids, combine:

- ✓ 1 cup of water
- ✓ 1 tablespoon of ACV

Drink 3x daily. You can start to see the relief supplied by this helpful combination within half an hour.

For topical relief, combine:
- ✓ ½ cup of water
- ✓ ½ cup ACV

Soak a cotton ball or soft towel within the mixture, and apply the mixture right to the affected area generally as needed, reducing inflammation and relieving the pain that results.

Relieve Insect Bites

Being bitten or stung by an insect can trip some reactions that may range between mildly uncomfortable to life-threatening. Some insect stings and bites aren't life-threatening, they can create skin conditions that itch, burn or sting, and will last all night, days, as well as weeks! Using apple cider vinegar is a healing treatment for bites you have and even to avoid long term bites! The naturally occurring acids and enzymes in apple cider vinegar become a deterrent against bugs that may bite and sting. In a position to detect the distasteful and aromatic components of ACV from afar, bugs are discouraged from even approaching a person who has ACV on your skin.

To produce a bug spray, combine inside a spray bottle:
- ✓ *1 cup of ACV*
- ✓ *½ cup of water*

Spray your skin using the mixture or make use of a towel to get the result on your skin and effectively deter bugs from stinging or biting.

To produce a localized treatment for soothing stings and bites, apply undiluted ACV to your skin using a towel or cotton ball every a quarter-hour. Not merely does this prevent inflammation at the source on the sting or bite; also, it helps to neutralize the venom excreted from the insect.

Do not hesitate to get immediate medical assistance if you believe your unique reaction warrants medical intervention.

Mitigate Jellyfish Stings

Few people know much about jellyfish stings or why they could be so agonizing. Jellyfish release nematocysts using their tentacles, which stick in your skin and release toxins into the bloodstream. These nematocysts could cause minor to excruciating pain, and they may warrant medical assistance in severe cases when breathing and vision are affected. Within the less extreme, but still unpleasant, cases of jellyfish stings, probably the most well-known treatment can be to use urine for the affected area.

Although some cases could find the use of urine effective in soothing the irritation that results from jellyfish stings, ACV is an all-natural option to urine that may soothe your skin by releasing the tentacles and delivering necessary nutrients to your skin for a quick repair. Apple cider vinegar has acetic acid that acts to soothe jellyfish stings in two ways:

1. Reducing inflammation, allowing the tentacles release from your skin and stopping the delivery in the toxins towards the sufferer's bloodstream.

2. Neutralizing the reaction within your skin, bloodstream, and nerves, relieving the pain with the sting promptly and effectively.

To produce a topical solution, apply undiluted ACV right to the site of the jellyfish sting.
Reapply as needed.

While you're even now experiencing pain, help to make *a glass or two by combining:*
- ✓ 1 tablespoon of ACV
- ✓ 1 cup of water

Drink once one hour for 4 hours to ease inflammation, deliver essential reparative minerals and vitamins to your skin, and help out with removing the poisons from the bloodstream and organs.

Decrease the Exposure to Facial "Masks"

Using a mix of apple cider vinegar along with other health-restoring products like a topical face mask shows to ease symptoms of skin irritation like redness, acne, and discolouration while improving the looks and quality of your skin. Assists in balancing the natural oil production of the skin (face and neck), apple cider vinegar's acetic and malic acids help out with unclogging pores and removing grime that may be deposited on the facial skin throughout the everyday routine. Assisting to restore a favorable pH balance to your skin, ACV shows drastic leads to acne sufferers'- reduced amount of irritation and incidence of pimples and blemishes on the skin.

Abundant with vitamin C and beta carotene, ACV's most impressive benefit may be the decrease in free radical harm to the skin over a cellular level, improving the fitness of your skin and preventing further skin surface damage that can be derived from contact with everyday waste like smoke, UV light, and polluting of the environment.

To produce a beneficial skin mask, mash the next ingredients right into a paste:

- ½ cup of ACV
- ½ of just one 1 avocado
- 1 tablespoon of natural, unprocessed, organic honey.

Apply right to your skin for 15-30 minutes, removing the mask by rinsing with hot water.

This specific mix contains rich levels of antioxidants, healthy fats, vitamins, minerals, and enzymes that absorb into the skin and help:

- Promote blood circulation, repair damage and restore skin health.
- Regulate pH and oil production.
- Remove dirt and germs through the skin's surface and pores.

Lessen Age Spots

Age spots are brown or tan oval-shaped discolorations on your skin that are derived from exposure to sunlight for extended periods. These hyperpigmented reactions normally develop in women and men older than forty, and may become darker and much more noticeable in the future. While there are chemical treatments and laser treatments designed to whiten these areas and better blend them with surrounding skin tones, many age spot sufferers choose to improve the appearance of their skin through more natural methods such as apple cider vinegar.

With ample amounts of vitamin C and beta carotene that act as powerful antioxidants, apple cider vinegar can assist in the repair of damaged skin cells. In addition to repairing the skin's cells, ACV also acts to regenerate the skin cells and improve the appearance of age spots by renewing the skin's surface.

To produce a topical aid, combine:

- ½ cup of ACV
- ½ cup of water

Apply to these spots on a towelette for thirty minutes 3 times per day.

Many have reported seeing dramatic improvements in the looks of age places following a few short weeks of the treatment.

Furthermore, you can even aid the body's reparative systems in regenerating skin cells and fighting free radical damage by drinking a regular ACV drink.

To produce a drink, combine:

- ✓ 1 cup of water
- ✓ 1 tablespoon of ACV

Drink daily.

Counteract Varicose Veins

Varicose veins are those bulging or discolored veins that may be combined with pain and sensitivity or just end up being an eyesore. Caused by pressure and a reduction in circulation to the affected area, varicose veins are most commonly in the legs, feet, and ankles. Some contributing factors to varicose veins are tight-fitting clothing, extended periods of standing or walking, and crossing the legs at the knee while sitting. To reduce the chances of developing varicose veins, you can:

- Wear less-restrictive clothing
- Improve your daily diet and remain hydrated
- Rub your feet and legs to boost circulation
- Prop up your feet while sitting to lessen the pressure positioned on the low extremities.

Another treatment that has shown to become quite helpful in alleviating varicose veins is apple cider vinegar. With blood-improving qualities that help detoxify and increase circulation, ACV can prevent circumstances that may aggravate the veins in the legs, ankles, and feet while also assisting in removing dead cells and arteries from the affected areas.

To produce a drink, combine within a blender:
- ✓ 1 cup of coconut milk
- ✓ 1 cup of strawberries (or kiwi or other tropical fruit)
- ✓ 1 tablespoon of ACV

Ice, as needed, Blend until desired consistency is achieved, and drink daily.

To produce a localized treatment, combine:
- ✓ ½ cup of water
- ✓ ½ cup of ACV

Soak a towel or washcloth using the mixture and apply right to veins for 20-30 minutes each time. This topical treatment helps to reduce inflammation of the skin and veins while also promoting circulation and blood flow on-site.

Manage Nail Fungus

Did you know apple cider vinegar acts as a highly effective treatment for fungus, as well as bacteria, viruses, and germs?

In a position to be studied orally or applied externally to be able to treat and stop fungal infections from the nails, ACV has unique uses and benefits that far outweigh those of prescriptions and over-the-counter medications.

ACV naturally delivers:

- Antifungal agents plus a selection of immunity-boosting vitamins.
- Minerals that help out with the reparation and healthy growth of nails.
- Antioxidants that help support preventing future fungal growth.

To produce a drink, combine:
- ✓ 1 cup of water
- ✓ 1 tablespoon of ACV

Drink daily for use as both cure and preventive measures.

ACV also has shown to be effective in killing fungus and restoring nail health when applied right to the source of fungal growth. The ACV seeps beneath the nail, penetrating from the nails' pores, and treats the encompassing nail bed.

To produce a nail soak, pour undiluted ACV right into a small bowl.

Allow nails rest there for 15-30 minutes at the same time almost every other hour before fungus subsides.

Cleanse and Push away Infection from Cuts

Probably the most dangerous consequence of a cut or abrasion is infection. After the skin continues to be opened, irritants like germs, bacteria, viruses, and fungi can seep into the bloodstream and cause infection at the site of the cut, as well as throughout the body. Cleaning the cut thoroughly with warm water and soap and covering the wound with a bandage are the two most essential and efficient preventive measures you can take to minimize the risk of infection.

The most beneficial steps to take to safeguard your health and the wound itself are to ensure that:

1. The wound remains free from foreign toxins

2. Your defence mechanisms are functioning properly

Apple cider vinegar can provide both these health-boosting benefits. It's filled with antiseptic, antiviral, and antibacterial properties. Apple cider vinegar would help fight any disease-fighting capability assailants that can be found, as well as safeguard the wound from any future germ exposure. ACV also includes powerful antioxidants that can help inside the regeneration of skin cells, improving the recovery process.

To produce a topical solution, combine:
- ✓ 1 tablespoon of water
- ✓ 1 tablespoon of ACV.

Following cleansing and ahead of within the wound, connect with the wound to provide additional protection against infection, and enhance the natural healing process. You can even drink ACV to optimize your disease fighting capability functioning and safeguard your wellbeing from germs that enter the site in the cut and travel through the bloodstream. Fighting free radicals and toxins within the blood, ACV has powerful vitamins, minerals, and nutrients that combine to combat immune system attackers effectively, leaving your body healthy and able to heal properly.

To Help Make The Drink, Combine:
- ✓ 1 cup of water
- ✓ 1 tablespoon of ACV.

Drink daily as the cut continues to be healing.

Produce Your Own Deodorant

Odour on your body can be the effect of a number of factors that range between sweat to bacteria, which is frequently strongest in parts of the body that can be restricted by clothing or creased, allowing moisture to stay (like the armpits) where bacteria can thrive. An alarming amount of people are unaware that they're placing chemical-laden, store-bought deodorants directly onto a thin layer of skin that covers lymph nodes and veins in the armpit. This highway of blood transporting veins and nodes absorbs the chemicals and additives in deodorants and antiperspirants, it delivers them throughout the body in the bloodstream.

As a result of the possibility of health hazards that can result from the chemicals used in these products, many consumers are opting for natural forms of deodorants that safely and effectively kill the cause of the odour without risking their health. *Apple cider vinegar can be used as an effective deodorant that does not pose health risks and boosts the body's overall health.*

To produce a homemade deodorant, combine:
- ✓ 1 tablespoon of water
- ✓ 1 tablespoon of ACV

Apply the mixture to the armpit or section of odour using a cotton ball and invite it to dry.

Not merely does this application kill odour-causing and infection-breeding bacteria, it is absorbed into the bloodstream. It helps to assist the body's everyday functioning by ensuring the systems through the entire body receive necessary nutrients.

To produce a preventive drink, combine:
- ✓ 1 cup of water

- ✓ 1 tablespoon of ACV

Drink daily to reap the advantages of health-boosting vitamins, minerals, and antioxidants that prevent odour-causing bacteria from breeding in the body and on the skin's surface.

Chapter 9
Side Effects of Apple Cider Vinegar

Whether consumed in the liquid or tablet form, Apple Cider Vinegar is ideal for treating many health issues. However, you should always understand that Apple Cider Vinegar is highly acidic in nature. While controlled intake has pH balancing effects, an excessive amount of consumption can imbalance the state of homeostasis inside our body. Some harmful effects that you should look out for are:

Reduced potassium levels

The acetic acid content of Apple Cider Vinegar in high quantity causes potassium deficiency which results in brittle and softer bones.

Digestive issues

No doubt, Apple Cider Vinegar is a superb remedy for acid reflux disorder. However, consuming an excessive amount causes diarrhea, heartburn, and indigestion.

Interactions with other medication

If you are currently taking insulin, laxatives, or any other, you have to check with your doctor before consuming Apple Cider Vinegar. It is because Apple Cider Vinegar may react with these medicines to get harmful effects on your body.

Damaged tooth enamel

Apple Cider Vinegar is saturated in its acidity. Consequently, you should never consume it directly. It's best that you utilize a straw or choose many diluted versions to keep the enamel of one's teeth. Prolonged contact with Apple Cider Vinegar could make the enamel weak and yellowish. You may even immediately brush your teeth soon after consuming to lessen the damage.

Chapter 10
How to Make ACV from Home

For quite some time, people have resorted to simple fermentation ways to produce wine in their homes. Now vinegar is a fancy French word for *"sour wine"*. So, if you're able to produce wine from home, you need to have the ability to get Apple Cider Vinegar in the home. The procedure is slightly time-consuming. However, the methodology details are incredibly satisfying. The approach to producing Apple Cider Vinegar from home isn't as hard as you imagine. *It is usually best recommended that you use organic apples to make your cider. Wash these apples (approximately 10 of them) and slice them into quarters. Let these slices rest at room temperature. As expected, they will turn brown. Put these brown apples in a glass jar and cover them with water. The level of water should be just enough to drown all the slices.*

Now, take a cheese-cloth and simply place it over the jar. You need not tie it or secure it as you need to allow oxygen *to enter the apples that have been soaked in the water. Now, find a warm place in your home and just place the whole apparatus as it is. This jar must be allowed to rest for at least six months. Make sure that you stir it at least once a week. After six months, take this jar down. You will notice the formation of a layer of scum at the surface of the jar.*

This is the result of the fermentation of the apples due to bacteria. The layer will almost look like bubbles that you see in a bucket of water when you throw in some soap and shake it.

The next step is to filter this liquid. Take a larger jar and place a cheesecloth over the jar containing the apples. This time, secure the cheesecloth tightly. Just tip the jar containing apples over the larger jar. The liquid will trickle through this into the second jar. Allow the entire liquid to be transferred into your larger jar.

Now, the new jar of liquid must be allowed to rest in a warm place. It should not be touched for at least four weeks. At the end of this long wait, you will have some beautiful amber colored apple cider vinegar that can be used for several home remedies.

The advantages of using homemade apple cider vinegar are numerous. Not merely are they far better in yielding results; also, they are purer forms that decrease the risks of side effects. Since you will be the one who managed to get, you will be sure of the hygiene and the cleanliness of the complete process. Of course, they could thoroughly test your patience in the first few times. However, if you can see the health benefits and can experience the joy of creating these exotic ingredients in your kitchen, it will all be worth it!

Precautions

Apple Cider Vinegar is undoubtedly the better product with regards to healing various ailments. However, we should ensure that the products are also consumed in the recommended amounts. They don't cause any harmful unwanted effects or health issues. However, an excessive amount could be disastrous. That is true for Apple Cider Vinegar.

CPSIA information can be obtained
at www.ICGtesting.com
Printed in the USA
BVHW070109240221
600901BV00006B/321